English for Biomedical Scientists

Ramón Ribes · Palma Iannarelli
Rafael F. Duarte

Ramón Ribes · Palma Iannarelli
Rafael F. Duarte

English for Biomedical Scientists

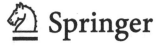 Springer

Ramón Ribes
Hospital Reina Sofia
Serv. Radiología
14005 Córdoba
Spain

Palma Iannarelli
University College London
Gower Street
London
United Kingdom WC1E 6BT

Rafael F. Duarte
Hospital Duran i Reynals
Inst. Català d'Oncologia
Servicio de Hematología Clinica
Av. Gan Via s/n km 2.7,
08907 Barcelona
Spain

ISBN 978-3-540-77126-5   ISBN 978-3-540-77127-2 (eBook)
DOI 10.1007/978-3-540-77127-2
Springer Dordrecht Heidelberg London New York

Library of Congress Control Number: 2009926060

Cover design: Estudio Calamar, F. Steinen-Broo, Pau/Girona, Spain

Printed on acid-free paper

Springer is part of Springer Science+Business Media (www.springer.com)

Preface

Biomedical scientists wishing to improve their capacity to communicate effectively in scientific English can find a great abundance of texts on the topic, from standard textbooks on English grammar to more practical manuals on scientific writing. Why then, you may wonder, would anyone want to write yet another book about scientific English? The quick answer is that our book is the first one to be aimed at a different group of readers. Other books on scientific English are written exclusively by and for native English speakers. Even the books that have added occasional chapters or appendixes for the benefit of international readers take for granted that their readership's mother tongue is English. The reality is that this is not the case for virtually all international biomedical scientists working in non-English-speaking countries. Even so, they still need to communicate in scientific English on many occasions. Nor is it the case for a very significant percentage of biomedical scientists at early stages in their career training and working at leading universities and research centers in English-speaking countries. Our book is directed at all those international scientists who, in addition to developing their scientific skills, have to face the additional challenge of communicating and being competitive in a language that is not their own. Our book shares with you more than ten years of first-hand experience in various areas associated with the use of English for biomedical scientists. We, the authors, have faced the very challenge that the book describes in our own professional experience.

The information contained in this book is as comprehensive as possible, but also presented in a practical, easy-to-read and understandable way with many examples. Some units cover somewhat more general topics on English grammar and English writing applied to biomedical sciences. Others deal with practical professional information such as résumé and cover-letter writing, attendance at international conferences, scientific presentations, or preparing for a successful job interview in English. Finally, there are units on technical aspects such as laboratory environment and writing, safety and biohazards, and animal work. This all-in-one comprehensive combination, with a focus on non-native-English-speaking scientists, makes this book unique.

We welcome your comments and suggestions, critical or otherwise. They will form the basis for an improved next edition of this book. Write to us at englishbiomedscientists@yahoo.com

Ramón Ribes
Palma Iannarelli
Rafael F. Duarte

Acknowledgments

We would like to thank Rafael Duarte-Lesmes for the cartoons in Units XI and XIII.

Contents

Unit III
Usual Mistakes Made by Scientistis Speaking and Writing in English

Unit IV
Writing a Manuscript

Unit V
Writing Scientific Correspondence

Unit VI
Attending a Scientific Course or Conference

Unit VII
Giving Presentations for Biomedical Scientists

Unit VIII
Chairing a Scientific Discussion

Unit IX
Curriculum Vitae, Cover Letters, and Other Professional Letters

Unit X
Getting Ready for a Job Interview in English

Unit XI
The Laboratory Environment

Unit XII
Laboratory Writing

Unit XIII
Laboratory Safety and Biohazards

Unit XIV
Laboratory Animal Work

Unit XV
Latin and Greek Terminology

Unit XVI
Acronyms and Abbreviations

Unit XVII
Conversation Survival Guide

Unit I Methodological Approach to English for Biomedical Scientists

Introduction

English is the global language of communication in all major scientific, medical and technological fields today. For biomedical sciences in particular, English has now become the norm for communicating and sharing scientific information. Therefore, biomedical scientists require not only scientific skills and expertise, but also the capacity to communicate effectively in scientific English.

The majority of non-English biomedical scientists would have normally studied English as a second language at some point during their training. They are likely to read English without major problems. This is as long as it is just reading silently to themselves (?). Reading aloud is a totally different issue. The real challenge commences when faced with the fact that in order to be part of the global biomedical scientific world, they will require to understand and to express themselves using professional English for international presentations and meetings. Although these challenges are common to doctors in many medical specialties, as seen in other books of this series, the case for biomedi cal scientists is even stronger. As a professional group, international biomedical scientists are very likely, actually they are almost expected, to move to a foreign laboratory at some point in their careers, most commonly to an English-speaking country, in order to continue professional training and career development. For this reason, their English needs go well beyond reading, writing, and presenting, to actually being capable of applying for jobs, writing résumés, facing job interviews in English, and settling into a new working environment in English. In addition to biomedical scientists, biomedical scientific English is becoming a common requirement for international medical doctors from nearly every medical or surgical specialty. Many medical doctors from a variety of specialties complete their clinical training with laboratory-based research training periods.

We believe that this book of the series has great potential to train biomedical scientists who need a good command of English for professional purposes. The practical approach of the various units from direct experience of the authors will surely reduce the anticipated stress of having to learn important matters directly "on the job," will boost self-confidence, and secure more efficient and productive communication from the start.

R. Ribes et al., *English for Biomedical Scientists*,
DOI: 10.1007/978-3-540-77127-2_1, © Springer-Verlag Berlin Heidelberg 2009

Your First Exercise in English for Biomedical Scientists

Let's do a simple exercise. Read the following two examples of biomedical scientific English:

> Combined stimulation with SCF and G-CSF leads to a complete phosphorylation of STAT3 on serine727, which is mediated by the phosphatidylinositol-3 kinase pathway, and leads to maximal STAT transcriptional activity and synergistic effect on cell proliferation.

If you are an international biomedical scientist, we are pretty confident that you have understood what you have just read. You may not understand every acronym if you are not specialized in cytokines and cell signaling, but overall you understand the sentence and are perfectly capable of translating it into your own language. Unfortunately, translation is not only useless but deleterious to your scientific English with regard to fluency.

If you try to read the paragraph in English out loud, you may encounter difficulties. For a start, it may feel natural to pronounce SCF or G-CSF just simply as S – C – F or G – C – S – F (spelling the letters out). But would you pronounce STAT3 as S – T – A – T – three, or would you rather say stat – three?

If a conversation on the sentence starts and the audience is waiting for your opinion, you may begin to sweat.

Check all the words you are not able to pronounce easily and look them up in the dictionary.

Ask an English-speaking colleague to read it aloud; try to write it; you will probably find some difficulty in writing certain words.

Now check the words you are not able to write properly and look them up in the dictionary.

Finally, try to have a conversation on the topic.

> August 1st, 2008 -- Postdoctoral Position in Neurodevelopmental Biology, Seattle, Washington. Postdoctoral position in the University of Washington in Seattle available for two years to study the role of TXUK and SOX molecules in brain development. Candidates must have a PhD in Neurosciences, molecular, cellular, developmental biology or related field. Basic cellular and molecular biology and microscopy skills required. Highly motivated, mature and responsible scientist committed to working in a competitive academic environment sought. Please send résumé, cover letter and 3 reference contacts to: George Chen, Department of Biology, University of Washington, Seattle WA 98195. E-mail: e_chen@u.washington.edu

Again, if you are an international scientist in search of a postdoctoral position in the field of neurodevelopmental biology in the USA, this looks as a very appealing opportunity. You can read the advertisement without problem. If you are in the field, you probably know about TXUK and SOX, and the rest of it seems pretty self-explanatory. Are there any words that you do not understand or know how to spell correctly? Check them up in the dictionary. Read it out loud. Not bad so far.

Now the next step of the exercise is to sit down in front of a computer and try to write your cover letter or letter of intent. I see…, not so easy any more, right? Is the page still blank? Let us give you a hint. A cover letter is a letter that you send along with your CV, and allows you to introduce yourself to the employer or evaluator and express your interest in the position that you are applying for. But in addition, it is really your brief opportunity to capture the recipient's attention and direct it towards the information on your CV that is of particular value for the post. So, it is a very important document in a job application. And since we are at it, what about your résumé? In addition to being a brief written account of your personal, educational, and professional qualifications and experience, your CV is your ticket to an interview. Are you ready to write a competitive CV in English that will get you that ticket to a job interview? If your page remains blank and you have not been able to put together these basic documents, you will certainly need to carry on reading this book.

Notice how many problems have been raised by just one small paragraph of scientific English. Our advice is, once you have diagnosed your actual level of biomedical scientific English:

- Do not get depressed if it is below your expectations.
- Keep doing these exercises with progressively longer paragraphs that belong to your scientific field.
- Arrange scientific sessions in your group or institution in English. A session once a week, for instance a journal club, might be a good starting point. The sessions will keep you, and your colleagues, in touch with your scientific English. You will notice that you feel much more confident talking to colleagues with a similar level of English than talking to your native English teacher, as you will feel better talking to non-native English-speaking biomedical scientists than talking to native English-speaking ones. In these sessions you can rehearse the performance of talks and lectures so that when you give a presentation at an international meeting it is not the first time it has been delivered.
- Follow the units of this book in whichever order you think suits your needs best. The book follows a logical structure (see below), but since you are already a scientist who knows some general English, you may want to take the units in a different order based on your experience or upcoming challenges.

Structure of the Book

In order to deal with various practical aspects of the professional use of English by non-native biomedical scientists, we have structured this book in seventeen units, including this introduction (Unit I). The logical order of the units goes from a general grammatical summary to more practical and specific tasks in English, written English first, spoken English later, and specific scientific English terminology at the end.

Units II and III provide you with general background on English grammar usage and usual mistakes made by non-native English-speaking biomedical scientists. Unless you have a sound knowledge of general English grammar, you should probably start with these two units to set a solid foundation for your work in the rest of the units.

Units IV and V leave introductions behind and dive in for the main general tasks that a scientist has to perform in English: delivering good scientific writing in English and being able to effectively write scientific correspondence. We will provide you with the tools to communicate with journal editors and reviewers in a formal manner, and with principles and many examples of scientific writing in English as a foreign language.

Units VI to VIII move away from writing English and on to putting spoken English into practice. Attending a scientific course or conference in English, making a scientific presentation in English, and chairing a scientific session in English are all important tasks you need to prepare for. Don't let your lack of fluency in day-to-day English undermine your ability to actively participate or chair a session in a scientific meeting, or to deliver a good or even great presentation. We will discuss in detail practical aspects, tips, and useful sentences that will help you succeed in this task.

Unit IX starts a second part of the book that focuses on the English needs of biomedical scientists that are planning to work in an English-speaking lab. Their needs go beyond adequately reading, writing, and presenting in occasional conferences, to actually making the transition into a new professional environment in English. This second part of the book will introduce issues related to this language transition, which are somewhat more specific in some units of this book for biomedical scientists. Such scientists will have to be able to apply for jobs and write résumés and personal statements in English (Unit IX). Even more, they will have to be able to confirm the good initial impression from their résumés and cover letters in job interviews that will be held in English, as the readers will review in Unit X.

As if all these tasks weren't enough, the transition also demands rapid acquaintance with the new working environment. Units XI through XIV are designed to provide the non-native biomedical scientist with enough prior knowledge of laboratory work in English, including the laboratory environment itself, laboratory writing in English, laboratory safety, and biohazards which you will be required to know and understand before you even start working, as well as specific aspects of laboratory animal work. This preparation will surely reduce the anticipated stress of having to learn important matters directly "on the job", will boost self-confidence, and secure more efficient and productive communication from the start.

Two additional units, XV and XVI, on classic terminology and acronyms, and Unit XVII, with a general conversation survival guide will complete the structure of the book.

UNIT II

UNIT II

Unit II   English Grammar Usage

The first chapters are probably the least read by most readers in general and scientists in particular, and in our opinion it is precisely in the first chapters that the most important information of a book is displayed. It is in its first chapters that the foundations of a book are laid, and many readers do not optimize the reading of a manual because they skip its fundamentals.

This is a vital chapter because unless you have a sound knowledge of English grammar you will be absolutely unable to speak English as is expected from a well-trained researcher. At your expected English level it is definitely not enough just to be understood; you must speak fluently and your command of the English language must allow you to communicate with your colleagues regardless of their nationality.

As you will see immediately, this grammar section is made up of scientific sentences, so at the same time that you revise, for instance, the passive voice, you will be reviewing how to say usual sentences in day-to-day English used in laboratories, such as "the scientist wears two pairs of latex gloves during a radioactive experiment in case one of them tears."

Tenses

Talking About the Present

Present Continuous

Present continuous shows an action that is happening in the present time at or around the moment of speaking.

Present simple of the verb *to be* + gerund of the verb: *am/are/is* ...-ing.

Study this example:

- It is 8:30 in the morning. Dr. Hudson is in his new car on his way to the laboratory.

  So: He *is driving* to the laboratory. He is driving to the laboratory means that he is driving now, at the time of speaking.

R. Ribes et al., *English for Biomedical Scientists*,
DOI: 10.1007/978-3-540-77127-2_2, © Springer-Verlag Berlin Heidelberg 2009

USES

To talk about:

- Something that is hapzpening at the time of speaking (i.e., now):
  - Dr. Hudson *is going* to the tissue culture room.
  - Dr. Smith's colleague *is performing* a PCR.

- Something that is happening around or close to the time of speaking, but not necessarily exactly at the time of speaking:
  - Jim and John are postdoctoral associates in Dr. Smith's laboratory and they are having lunch in the cafeteria. John says: "I *am writing* an interesting article on origins of oligodendrocytes in the spinal cord. I'll give you a copy when I've finished writing it". As you can see John is not writing the article at the time of speaking. He means that he has begun to write the article but has not finished it yet. He is in the middle of writing it.

- Something that is happening for a limited period of time around the present (e.g., today, this week, this season, this year ...):
  - Our PhD students *are working* hard this term.

- Changing situations:
  - Scientists *are getting* closer to understanding how the brain works.

- Temporary situations:
  - I *am living* with other students until I can buy my own apartment.
  - I *am doing* a rotation in Dr. Thomson's laboratory until the end ofM ay.

Special use: Present continuous with a future meaning
In the following examples doing these things is already arranged.

- To talk about what you have arranged to do in the near future (personala rrangements).
  - We *are going* to the Neuroscience conference in London this month.
  - I *am having* dinner with a Nobel Prize scientist from Edinburgh tomorrow.

We do not use the simple present or *will* for personal arrangements.

Simple Present

Simple present shows an action that happens again and again (repeated action) in the present time, but not necessarily at the time of speaking.

FORM

The simple present has the following forms:

- Affirmative (remember to add -s or -es to the third person singular)

- Negative
  - I/we/you/they don't ...
  - He/she/it doesn't ...

- Interrogative
  - Do I/we/you/they ... ?
  - Does he/she/it ... ?

Study this example:

- Dr. Allan is the chairman of the Cancer Biology Department. He is at an international course in Greece at this moment.

So: He *is not running* the Cancer Biology Department now (because he is in Greece), but *he runs* the Cancer Biology Department.

USES

- To talk about something that happens all the time or repeatedly or something that is true in general. Here it is not important whether the action is happening at the time of speaking:
  - I *do* research using live animals.
  - Animal technicians *take care* of animals that are used in research.
  - For in situ hybridization experiments, all solutions *are* RNase-free.

- To say how often we do things:
  - I *start* my experiments at 9:30 every morning.
  - Dr. Taylor *teaches* biology twice a week.
  - How often *do you go* to an international stem cell course? Once a year.

- For a permanent situation (a situation that stays the same for a long time):
  - I *work* as a research assistant in the Cancer Biology department at Harvard Medical School. I have been working there for ten years.

- Some verbs are used only in simple tenses. These verbs are verbs of thinking or mental activity, feeling, possession and perception, and reporting verbs. We often use *can* instead of the present tense with verbs of perception:
  - I *can understand* now why the microscope is in such a bad condition.
  - I *can see* now the solution to the diagnostic problem.

- The simple present is often used with adverbs of frequency such as *always, often, sometimes, rarely, never, every week*, and *twice a year*:
  - PhD students *always* work very hard.
  - We *have* a lab meeting *every week*.

- Simple present with a future meaning. We use it to talk about timetables, schedules...
  - What time *does* the lab safety course *start*? It *starts* at 9.30.

Talking About the Future

Going To

<table>
<tr>
<td rowspan="1">USES</td>
<td>

• To say what we have already decided to do or what we intend to do in the future (do not use *will* in this situation):
  - I *am going to* attend the 40th annual meeting of the Society for Neuroscience next month.
  - There is a stem cell course in Boston next fall. *Are you going to* attend it?

• To say what someone has arranged to do (personal arrangements), but remember that we prefer to use the present continuous because it sounds more natural:
  - What time *are you going to meet* the Administrative Director?
  - What time *are you going to* begin the PCR?

• To say what we think will happen (making predictions):
  - The animals are agitated. I think we *are not going to* get good quality results.
  - We think this new technology *is going to* improve cloning efficiency in rodents.

• If we want to say what someone intended to do in the past but did not do, we use *was/were going to*:
  - He *was going to* do a PCR on the sample but finally changed his mind and decided to do a Southern Blot.

• To talk about past predictions we use *was/were going to*:
  - The research assistant had the feeling that the animal *was going to* suffer an allergic reaction to the anesthetic drug.

</td>
</tr>
</table>

Simple Future (Will)

<table>
<tr>
<td rowspan="1">FORM</td>
<td>

I/We *will* or *shall* (*will* is more common than *shall*. *Shall* is often used in questions to make offers and suggestions):

• *Shall* we go to the journal club next week? Oh, great idea!
• *Shall* I order more flasks for the laboratory?
• What *shall* we do now?

You/he/she/it/they *will*.
Negative: *shan't, won't*.

</td>
</tr>
</table>

USES

- We use *will* when we decide to do something at the time of speaking (remember that in this situation, you cannot use the simple present):
  - Have you finished the experiment?
  - No, I haven't had time to do it.
  - OK, don't worry, I *will* do it.

- When offering, agreeing, refusing, and promising to do something, or when asking someone to do something:
  - That experiment looks difficult for you. Do not worry, I **will** help you out.
  - Can I have the book about embryonic stem cells that I lent to you? Of course. I *will* give it back to you tomorrow.
  - Don't ask to use the confocal microscope without supervision. Dr. Harris *won't* allow you to.
  - I promise I *will* send you a copy of the latest article on molecular immunology as soon as I get it.
  - *Will* you help me out with this time-lapse experiment, please?

You do not use *will* to say what someone has already decided to do or arranged to do (remember that in this situation we use *going to* or the present continuous).

- To predict a future happening or a future situation:
  - Scientific research *will* find a cure for ALS.
  - Treatments for cancer *won't* be the same in the next two decades.

Remember that if there is something in the present situation that shows us what will happen in the future (near future) we use *going to* instead of *will*.

- With expressions such as: *probably, I am sure, I bet, I think, I suppose, I guess*:
  - I *will probably* attend the International Symposium.
  - You should listen to Dr. Helms giving a conference. I am *sure* you *will* love it.
  - I bet the animal *will* recover satisfactorily after the brain surgery.
  - I *guess* I *will* see you at the next annual meeting.

Future Continuous

FORM

Will be + gerund of the verb.

USES	

	• To say that we will be in the middle of something at a certain time in the future:
	  – This time tomorrow morning I *will be performing* my first PCR.
	
	• To talk about things that are already planned or decided (similar to the present continuous with a future meaning):
	  – I *will be making* no decisions tonight about the prospective employees.
	
	• To ask about people's plans, especially when we want something or want someone to do something (interrogative form):
	  – *Will* you *be helping* me mark the laboratory reports this evening?

Future Perfect

FORM	

	Will have + past participle of the verb.
	• To say that something will already have happened before a certain time in the future:
	  – I think the student *will* already *have arrived* by the time we begin the PCR.
	  – Next spring I *will have been working* for 25 years in the Cancer Biology Department of this institution.

Talking About the Past

Simple Past

FORM	

	The simple past has the following forms:
	• Affirmative:
	  – The past of the regular verbs is formed by adding *-ed* to the infinitive.
	  – The past of the irregular verbs has its own form.
	
	• Negative:
	  – *Did/didn't* + the base form of the verb.
	
	• Questions:
	  – *Did I/you/* ... + the base form of the verb.

USES	• To talk about actions or situations in the past (they have already finished):
	  − I really *enjoyed* the Institute's Christmas party very much.
	  − When I *worked* as an animal care technician in London, I *performed* a vasectomy on thirty male mice.
	
	• To say that one thing happened after another:
	  − Yesterday, I *was* walking towards the Molecular Genetics Department when I *saw* Dr Harris. So, I *stopped* and we *had* a chat about gene therapy and then we *went* to the canteen and *had* lunch together.
	
	• To ask or say *when* or *what time* something happened:
	  − When *were* you last on call?
	
	• To tell a story and to talk about happenings and actions that are not connected with the present (historical events):
	  − Alexander Fleming *discovered* penicillin.

Past Continuous

FORM	*Was/were* + gerund of the verb.

USES	• To say that someone was in the middle of doing something at a certain time. The action or situation had already started before this time but hadn't finished: • This time last year I *was writing* the article on contrast-enhanced MRI features of ankylosing spondylitis that has been recently published. Notice that the past continuous does not tell us whether an action was finished or not. Perhaps it was, perhaps it was not. • To describe a scene: • A lot of patients *were waiting* in the corridor to see a doctor.

Present Perfect

FORM	*Have/has* + past participle of the verb.

- To talk about the present result of a past action.
- To talk about a recent happening.

In the latter situation you can use the present perfect with the following particles:

- *Just* (i.e., a short time ago): to say something has happened a short time ago:
  - Dr. Ho *has just arrived* at the hospital. He is our new pediatric oncologist.

- *Already*: to say something has happened sooner than expected:
  - The second-year PhD student *has already finished* her presentation.

Remember that to talk about a recent happening we can also use the simple past:

- To talk about a period of time that continues up to the present (an unfinished period of time):
  - We use the expressions: *today, this morning, this evening, this week …*
  - We often use *ever* and *never*.

- To talk about something that we are expecting. In this situation we use *yet* to show that the speaker is expecting something to happen, but only in questions and negative sentences:
  - Dr. Helms *has not arrived yet*.

- To talk about something you have never done or something you have not done during a period of time that continues up to the present:
  - I *have not performed* a PCR since I was a post-doc.

- To talk about how much we have done, how many things we have done, or how many times we have done something:
  - I *have reported* that regional brain perfusion scan twice because the first report was lost.
  - Dr. Yimou *has performed* twenty tail biopsies this week.

- To talk about situations that exists for a long time, especially if we say *always*. In this case the situation still exists now:
  - Embryonic stem cells *have always been* a controversial issue.
  - Dr. Olmedo *has always been* a very talented scientist.

We also use the present perfect with these expressions:

- Superlative: *It is the most …*:
  - This is *the most* bizarre result I *have ever gotten*.
  - She is *the most* convincing speaker I *have ever heard*.

- The *first* (*second, third …*) *time …*:
  - This is the *first time* that I *have seen* a CT of a vertebral hemangiopericytoma.

Present Perfect Continuous

Shows an action that began in the past and has gone on up to the present time.

FORM	*Have/has been* + gerund.

USES	<ul><li>To talk about an action that began in the past and has recently stopped or just stopped: – You look tired. *Have you been working* all night? – No, *I have been writing* an article on the embryonic origins of motor neurons.</li><li>To ask or say how long something has been happening. In this case the action or situation began in the past and is still happening or has just stopped. – Dr. Sancho and Dr. Martos *have been working* together on the project *from* the beginning.</li></ul>We use the following particles:<ul><li>*How long* ...? (to ask how long): – *How long* have you been working as a research technician?</li><li>*For, since* (to say how long): – I have been working *for* ten years. – I have been working very hard *since* I got this grant.</li><li>*For* (to say how long as a period of time): – I have been generating transgenic animals *for* three years.</li></ul>Do not use *for* in expressions with *all*: "I have been working as a scientist *all* my life" (not "*for all* my life").<ul><li>*Since* (to say the beginning of a period): – I have been teaching biology *since* 1991.</li></ul>In the present perfect continuous the important thing is the action itself and it does not matter whether the action is finished or not. The action can be finished (just finished) or not (still happening). In the present perfect the important thing is the result of the action and not the action itself. The action is completely finished.

Past Perfect

Shows an action that happened in the past before another past action. It is the past of the present perfect.

FORM	*Had* + past participle of the verb.

USES	• To say that something had already happened before something else happened: – When I arrived at the vivarium, the animal technician *had* already *begun* microinjecting DNA constructs into the pronuclei of zygotes.

Past Perfect Continuous

Shows an action that began in the past and went on up to a time in the past. It is the past of the present perfect continuous.

FORM	*Had been* + gerund of the verb.

USES	• To say how long something had been happening before something else happened: – She *had been working* as a scientist for forty years before she was awarded the Nobel Prize.

Subjunctive

Imagine this situation:

- The scientist says to the technician, "Why don't you do a PCR on the samples we received today?"
- The scientist proposes (that) the technician do a PCR on the samples they received today.

The subjunctive is always formed with the base form of the verb (the infinitive without to):

- I suggest (that) you *work* harder.
- She recommended (that) he *give up* smoking while dictating.
- He insisted (that) she *perform a PCR on the samples* as soon as possible.
- He demanded (that) the research assistant *treat him* more politely.

Note that the subjunctive of the verb *to be* is usually passive:

- He insisted (that) the project proposal *be written* immediately.

You can use the subjunctive after:

- Proposing
- Suggesting
- Recommending
- Insisting
- Demanding

You can use the subjunctive for the past, present, or future:

- He *suggested* (that) the student *change* the format of the report.
- He *recommends* (that) his workers *give up* smoking.

Should is sometimes used instead of the subjunctive:

- The doctor recommended that *I should have* an MRI examination; he suspects that my meniscus is probably torn.

Wish, If Only, Would

Wish
- *Wish* + simple past. To say that we regret something (i.e., that something is not as we would like it to be) in the present:
  - *I wish I spoke* English well (but I cannot speak English well).
  - *I wish I lived* in Canada (but I don't live Canada).

- *Wish* + past perfect. To say that we regret something that happened or didn't happen in the past:
  - *I wish he hadn't treated his coworkers so badly* (but he treated his coworkers badly).
  - *I wish I hadn't worked* with her (but you did work with her).

- *Wish* + *would* + infinitive without *to* when we want something to happen or change or somebody to do something:
  - *I wish you wouldn't dictate* so slowly (note that the speaker is complaining about the present situation or the way people do things).
  - *I wish it would stop raining* (but it is still raining).

If Only
If only can be used in exactly the same way as *wish*. It has the same meaning as *wish* but is more dramatic:

- *If only* + past simple (expresses regret in the present):
  - *If only I spoke* English well.
  - *If only I lived* in Canada.

- *If only* + past perfect (expresses regret in the past):
  - *If only he hadn't treated* the patient's family so badly.
  - *If only I hadn't worked* with her.

After *wish* and *if only* we use *were* (with *I*, *he*, *she*, *it*) instead of *was*, and we do not normally use *would*, although sometimes it is possible, or *would have*.

When referring to the present or future, *wish* and *if only* are followed by a past tense, and when referring to the past by a past perfect tense.

Would

Would is used:

- As a modal verb in offers, invitations and requests (i.e., to ask someone to do something):
  - *Would* you help me to write an article on developmental origin of adipocytes? (request).
  - *Would* you like to come to the students' party tonight? (offer and invitation).
- After *wish* (see *Wish*).
- In *if* sentences (see *Conditionals*).
- Sometimes as the past of *will* (in reported speech):
  - Lidia said, "I will come to the lab tomorrow."
  - Lidia said that she *would* come to the lab tomorrow.
- When you remember things that often happened (similar to *used to*):
  - Isaac *used to* walk to work every day.
  - Isaac *would* walk to work every day.

Modal Verbs

FORM	- A modal verb always has the same form. - There is no *-s* ending in the third person singular, no *-ing* form and no *-edf* orm. - After a modal verb we use the infinitive without *to* (i.e., the base form of the verb).

These are the English modal verbs:

- *Can* (past form is *could*)
- *Could* (also a modal with its own meaning)
- *May* (past form is *might*)
- *Might* (also a modal with its own meaning)
- *Will*
- *Would*
- *Shall*
- *Should*
- *Ought to*
- *Must*
- *Need*
- *Dare*

FORM	We use modal verbs to talk about: • Ability • Necessity • Possibility • Certainty • Permission • Obligation

Expressing Ability

To express ability we can use:

- *Can* (only in the present tense)
- *Could* (only in the past tense)
- *Be able to* (in all tenses)

Ability in the Present

Can (more usual) or *am/is/are able to* (less usual):

- Claudio *can* generate transgenic mice.
- Claudio *is able to* generate transgenic mice.
- *Can* you speak English? Yes, I *can*.
- *Are you able to* speak English? Yes, I am.

Ability in the Past

Could (past form of *can*) or *was/were able to*.

We use *could* to say that someone had the *general* ability to do something:

- When I was an undergraduate student I *could* speak German.

We use *was/were able to* to say that someone managed to do something in one particular situation (*specific* ability to do something):

- Adriano *was able to* extract good quality RNA from the tissue samples.

Managed to can replace *was able to*:

- Adriano *managed to* extract good quality RNA from the tissue samples.

We use *could have* to say that we had the ability to do something but we didn't do it:

- He *could have* been a medical doctor but he became a scientist instead.

Sometimes we use *could* to talk about ability in a situation which we are imagining (here *could* = *would be able to*):

- I *couldn't* do your job. I'm not clever enough.

We use *will be able to* to talk about ability with a future meaning:

- If you keep on studying English you *will be able to* write articles for *Science* very soon.

Expressing Necessity

Necessity means that you cannot avoid doing something.

To say that it is necessary to do something we can use *must* or *have to*.

- Necessity in the present: *must, have/has to*.
- Necessity in the past: *had to*.
- Necessity in the future: *must* or *will have to*.

Notice that to express necessity in the past we do not use *must*.

There are some differences between *must* and *have to*:

- We use *must* when the speaker is expressing personal feelings or authority, saying what he or she thinks is necessary:
  - Your chest X-ray film shows severe emphysema. You *must* give up smoking.
- We use *have to* when the speaker is not expressing personal feelings or authority. The speaker is just giving facts or expressing the authority of another person (external authority), often a law or a rule:
  - All researchers *have to* keep a record of their work in a formal notebook.

If we want to express that there is necessity to avoid doing something, we use *mustn't* (i.e., *not allowed to*):

- You *mustn't* eat anything before the intravenous administration of contrast agent.

Expressing No Necessity

To express that there is no necessity we can use the negative forms of *need* or *have to*:

- No necessity in the present: *needn't* or *don't/doesn't have to*.
- No necessity in the past: *didn't need, didn't have to*.
- No necessity in the future: *won't have to*.

Notice that "there is no necessity to do something" is completely different from "there is a necessity not to do something".

In conclusion, we use *mustn't* when we are not allowed to do something or when there is a necessity not to do it, and we use the negative form of *have to* or *needn't* when there is no necessity to do something but we can do it if we want to:

- The doctor says *I mustn't* get overtired before the procedure but *I needn't* stay inb ed.
- The doctor says *I mustn't* get overtired before the procedure but *I don't have to* stay in bed.

Expressing Possibility

To express possibility we can use *can, could, may,* or *might* (from more to less certainty: can → may → might → could).

But also note that "can" is used of ability (or capacity) to do something; "may" of permission or sanction to do it.

Possibility in the Present

To say that something is possible we use *can, may, might, could*:

- High doses of radiation *can* cause you to get cancer (high level of certainty).
- Radiation *may* actually cause you to get cancer (moderate to high level of certainty).
- Radiation *might* cause you to get thyroid cancer (moderate to low level of certainty).
- Radiation *could* cause you to get bone cancer (low level of certainty).

Possibility in the Past

To say that something was possible in the past we use *may have, might have, could have*:

- The lesion *might have* been detected on CT if the slice thickness had been thinner.

Could have is also used to say that something was a possibility or opportunity but it didn't happen:

- That experiment you performed was dangerous. You *could have* died.

I *couldn't have* done something (i.e., I wouldn't have been able to do it if I had wanted or tried to do it):

- She *couldn't have* seen the size difference between the DNA fragments, because the resolution of the gel was poor.

Possibility in the Future

To talk about possible future actions or happenings we use *may, might, could* (especially in suggestions):

- I don't know where to do my next postdoctoral position. I *may/might go* to the States.
- Dr. Sirolli said we *could* go to the neuroscience meeting.

When we are talking about possible future plans we can also use the continuous form *may/might/could be + -ing* form:

- I *could be going* to the next safety meeting.

Expressing Certainty

To say we are sure that something is true we use *must*:

- You have been working in the lab all night. You *must* be very tired (i.e., I am sure that you are tired).

To say that we think something is impossible we use *can't*:

- According to his clinical laboratory results, that diagnosis *can't* be true (i.e., it is impossible that that diagnosis is true *or* I am sure that that diagnosis is not true).

For past situations we use *must have* and *can't have*. We can also use *couldn't have* instead of *can't have*:

- Taking into consideration the situation, the family of the patient *couldn't have* asked for more.

Remember that to express certainty we can also use *will*:

- I *will* be back in the lab in five minutes.
- Laboratory safety procedures *will* vary from facility to facility.

Expressing Permission

To talk about permission we can use *can, may* (more formal than *can*), or *be allowed to*.

Permission in the Present

Can, may, or *am/is/are allowed to*:

- You *can* smoke if you like.
- You *are allowed to* smoke.
- You *may* attend the Symposium.

Permission in the Past

Was/were allowed to:

- *Were you allowed to* go into the interventional radiology suite without surgical scrubs?

Permission in the Future

Will be allowed to:

- You *will be allowed to* work in the UK if you have a work permit.

To ask for permission we use *can, may, could*, or *might* (from less to more formal) but not *be allowed to*:

- Hi Hannah, *can* I borrow your digital camera? (if you are asking for a friend's digital camera).
- Dr. Ho, *may* I borrow your digital camera? (if you are talking to an acquaintance).
- *Could* I use your digital camera, Dr. Coltrane? (if you are talking to a colleague you do not know at all).
- *Might* I use your digital camera, Dr. De Roos? (if you are asking for the chairman's digital camera).

Expressing Obligation or Giving Advice

Obligation means that something is the right thing to do.

When we want to say what we think is a good thing to do or the right thing to do we use *should* or *ought to* (a little stronger than *should*).

Should and *ought to* can be used for giving advice:

- You *ought to* sleep more.
- You *should* work out.
- You *ought to* give up smoking.
- *Should* he see a doctor? Yes, I think he should.
- When *should* we leave the lab? We should leave in 5 minutes.

Conditionals

Conditional sentences have two parts:

1. "If-clause"
2. Main clause

In the sentence "If I were you, I would go to the annual meeting of the American Society of Hematology", "If I were you" is the if-clause, and "I would go to the annual meeting of the American Society of Hematology" is the main clause.

If we receive the research grant, we can hire more research assistants.

The if-clause can come before or after the main clause. We often put a comma when the if-clause comes first.

Main Types of Conditional Sentences

Type 0

To talk about things that always are true (general truths).

If + simple present + simple present:

- *If* you expose your skin to phenol, you get a skin burn.
- *If* you drink too much alcohol, you get a sore head.
- *If* you take drugs habitually, you become addicted.
- Ice melts *if* the temperature is above 0 degrees Celsius.

Note that the examples above refer to things that are normally true. They make no reference to the future; they represent a present simple concept. This is the basic (or classic) form of the conditional type 0.

There are possible variations of this form. In the if-clause and in the main clause we can use the present continuous, present perfect simple, or present perfect continuous instead of the present simple. In the main clause we can also use the imperative instead of the present simple:

- Students only get a certificate *if* they *have attended* the course regularly.

So the type 0 form can be reduced to:

- *If* + present form + present form or imperative.

Present forms include the present simple, present continuous, present perfect simple, and present perfect continuous.

Type 1

To talk about future situations that the speaker thinks are likely to happen (the speaker is thinking about a real possibility in the future).

If + simple present + future simple (*will*):

- *If* I find something new about the treatment of malignant obstructive jaundice, I will tell you.
- *If* we find out how motor neurons die in people with ALS, we will be able to design treatments to prevent this from happening.

These examples refer to future things that are possible and it is quite probable that they will happen. This is the basic (or classic) form of the conditional type 1.

There are possible variations of the basic form. In the if-clause we can use the present continuous, the present perfect, or the present perfect continuous instead of the present simple. In the main clause we can use the future continuous, future perfect simple, or future perfect continuous instead of the future simple. Modals such as *can*, *may*, or *might* are also possible.

So the form of type 1 can be reduced to:

- *If* + present form + future form

Future forms include the future simple, future continuous, future perfect simple, and future perfect continuous.

Type 2

To talk about future situations that the speaker thinks are possible but not probable (the speaker is imagining a possible future situation) or to talk about unreal situations in the present.

If + simple past + conditional (*would*):

- Peter, *if* you *worked* harder, you *would* be finished with your studies.
- *If* I *were* you, I *would* go to the Annual Meeting of the American Society of Hematology (but I am not you).
- *If* I *were* a resident again, I *would* go to Harvard Medical School for a whole year to complete my training period (but I am not a resident).

There are possible variations of the basic form. In the if-clause we can use the past continuous instead of the past simple. In the main clause we can use *could* or *might* instead of *would*.

So the form of type 2 can be reduced to:

- *If* + past simple or continuous + *would*, *could*, or *might*.

Type 3

To talk about past situations that didn't happen (impossible actions in the past).

If + past perfect + perfect conditional (*would have*):

- *If* he *had* been in the lab when the explosion occurred, it *would have* injured him
- *If* she *had* missed her flight, he *would have* been waiting for her at the airport forh ours.

As you can see, we are talking about the past.

This is the basic (or classic) form of the third type of conditional. There are possible variations. In the if-clause we can use the past perfect continuous instead of the past perfect simple. In the main clause we can use the continuous form of the perfect conditional instead of the perfect conditional simple. *Would probably*, *could*, or *might* instead of *would* are also possible (when we are not sure about something).

In Case

"The scientist wears two pairs of latex gloves during a radioactive experiment *in case* one of them tears." *In case one of them tears* because it is possible that one of them tears during the experiment (in the future).

Note that we don't use *will* after *in case*. We use a present tense after *in case* when we are talking about the future.

In case is not the same as *if*. Compare these sentences:

- We'll buy some more food and drink *if* the new residents come to our department's party. (Perhaps the new residents will come to our party. If they come, we will buy some more food and drink; if they don't come, we won't.)
- We will buy some food and drink *in case* the new residents come to our department's party. (Perhaps the new residents will come to our department's party. We will buy some more food and drink whether they come or not.)

We can also use *in case* to say why someone did something in the past:

- He rang the bell again *in case* the nurse hadn't heard it the first time. (Because it was possible that the nurse hadn't heard it the first time.)

In case of (= if there is):

- *In case of* pregnancy, avoid work with radioactive materials.

Unless

"Don't take these pills *unless* you are extremely anxious." (Don't take these pills except if you are extremely anxious.) This sentence means that you can take the pills only if you are extremely anxious.

We use *unless* to make an exception to something we say. In the example above the exception is *you are extremely anxious*.

We often use *unless* in warnings:

- *Unless* you send the application form today, you won't be considered for the MRC New Investigator Research grant.

It is also possible to use *if* in a negative sentence instead of *unless*:

- Don't take those pills *if you aren't* extremely anxious.
- *If you don't send* the application form today, you won't be considered for the MRC New Investigator Research grant.

As Long As, Provided (That), Providing (That)

These expressions mean *but only if*:

- You can use my new pen to sign your report *as long as* you write carefully (i.e., *but only if* you write carefully).
- Going by car to the institute is convenient *provided* (*that*) you have somewhere to park (i.e., *but only if* you have somewhere to park).
- *Providing* (*that*) she studies the clinical cases, she will deliver a bright presentation.

Passive Voice

Study these examples:

- The laboratory was destroyed by a big fire (passive).
- A big fire destroyed the laboratory (active).

Both sentences are correct and mean the same. They are two different ways of saying the same thing, but in the passive sentence we try to make the object of the active sentence ("a big fire") more important by putting it at the beginning. So, we prefer to use the passive when it is not that important who or what did the action. In the example above, it is not so important how the laboratory was destroyed.

Active sentence:

- Fleming (subject) discovered (active verb) penicillin (object) in 1950.

Passive sentence:

- Penicillin (subject) was discovered (passive verb) by Fleming (agent) in 1950.

The passive verb is formed by putting the verb *to be* into the same tense as the active verb and adding the past participle of the active verb:

- Discovered (active verb) – was discovered (*be* + past participle of the active verb).

The object of an active verb becomes the subject of the passive verb ("penicillin"). The subject of an active verb becomes the agent of the passive verb ("Fleming"). We can leave out the agent if it is not important to mention it or we don't know it. If we want to mention it, we will put it at the end of the sentence preceded by the particle *by* ("… by Fleming").

Some sentences have two objects, indirect and direct. In these sentences the passive subject can be either the direct object or the indirect object of the active sentence:

- The veterinarian gave the research animals a new treatment.

There are two possibilities:

- A new treatment was given to the research animals.
- The research animals were given a new treatment.

Passive Forms of Present and Past Tenses

In the examples below we use the verb *write*. This is an irregular verb, therefore it does not end in – *ed* in the past tense. Write (present), wrote (past), written (past participle).

Simple Present

Active:
- Dr. Di Prata writes a paper on stem cells.

Passive:
- A paper on stem cells is written by Dr. Di Prata.

Simple Past

Active:
- Dr. Di Prata wrote a paper on stem cells.

Passive:
- A paper on stem cells was written by Dr. Di Prata.

Present Continuous

Active:
- Dr. Di Prata is writing a paper on stem cells.

Passive:
- A paper on stem cells is being written by Dr. Di Prata.

Past Continuous

Active:
- Dr. Di Prata was writing a paper on stem cells.

Passive:

- A paper on stem cells was being written by Dr. Di Prata.

Present Perfect

Active:

- Dr. Di Prata has written a paper on stem cells.

Passive:

- A paper on stem cells has been written by Dr. Di Prata.

Past Perfect

Active:

- Dr. Di Prata had written a paper on stem cells.

Passive:

- A paper on stem cells had been written by Dr. Di Prata.

In sentences of the type "people say/consider/know/think/believe/expect/understand ... that ...", such as "Doctors consider that AIDS is a fatal disease", we have two possible passive forms:

- AIDS is considered to be a fatal disease.
- It is considered that AIDS is a fatal disease.

Have/Get Something Done

> **FORM**
>
> *Have/get* + object + past participle.

Get is a little more informal than *have*, and it is often used in informal spoken English:

- You should *get* the ultracentrifuge machine fixed.
- You should *have* the ultracentrifuge machine fixed.

When we want to say that we don't want to do something ourselves and we arrange for someone to do it for us, we use the expression *have something done*:

- The patient had all his metal objects removed in order to prevent accidents during the MR examination.

Sometimes the expression *have something done* has a different meaning:

- John had his knee broken playing a football match. MRI showed a meniscal tear.

It is obvious that this doesn't mean that he arranged for somebody to break his knee. With this meaning, we use *have something done* to say that something (often something not nice) happened to someone.

Supposed To

Supposed to can be used in the following ways:

Can be used like *said to*:

- The chairman is supposed to be the one who runs the department.

To say what is planned or arranged (and this is often different from what really happens):

- The fourth year resident is supposed to read this CT.

To say what is not allowed or not advisable:

- You are not supposed to drink alcohol while you are pregnant.

Reported Speech

Imagine that you want to tell someone else what the patient said. You can either repeat the patient's words or use reported speech.

The reporting verb (*said* in the examples below) can come before or after the reported clause (*there was a conference about stem cells that evening*), but it usually comes before the reported clause. When the reporting verb comes before, we can use *that* to introduce the reported clause or we can leave it out (leaving it out is more informal). When the reporting verb comes after, we cannot use *that* to introduce the reported clause.

The reporting verb can report statements and thoughts, questions, orders, and requests. Here are a few commonly used reporting verbs: *admit, advise, ask, deny, explain, promise, reply, say, tell, warn.*

Reporting in the Present

When the reporting verb is in the present tense, it isn't necessary to change the tense of the verb:

- "I'll help you guys with this maxiprep", he says.
- He says (that) he will help us with this maxiprep.
- "The administration of BrdU and tissue preparation will take place this afternoon", he says.

- He says (that) the administration of BrdU and tissue preparation will take place this afternoon.

Reporting in the Past

When the reporting verb is in the past tense, the verb in direct speech usually changes in the following ways:

- Simple present changes to simple past.
- Present continuous changes to past continuous.
- Simple past changes to past perfect.
- Past continuous changes to past perfect continuous.
- Present perfect changes to past perfect.
- Present perfect continuous changes to past perfect continuous.
- Past perfect stays the same.
- Future changes to conditional.
- Future continuous changes to conditional continuous.
- Future perfect changes to conditional perfect.
- Conditional stays the same.
- Present forms of modal verbs stay the same.
- Past forms of modal verbs stay the same.

Pronouns, adjectives, and adverbs also change. Here are some examples:

- First person singular changes to third person singular.
- Second person singular changes to first person singular.
- First person plural changes to third person plural.
- Second person plural changes to first person plural.
- Third person singular changes to third person plural.
- Now changes to then.
- Today changes to that day.
- Tomorrow changes to the day after.
- Yesterday changes to the day before.
- This changes to that.
- Here changes to there.
- Ago changes to before.

It is not always necessary to change the verb when you use reported speech. If you are reporting something and you feel that it is still true, you do not need to change the tense of the verb, but if you want you can do it:

- The treatment of choice for severe urticaria after intravenous contrast administration is epinephrine.
- He said (that) the treatment of choice for severe urticaria after intravenous contrast administration is epinephrine.

or

- He said (that) the treatment of choice for severe urticaria after intravenous contrast administration was epinephrine.

Reporting Questions

Yes and No Questions

We use *whether* or *if*:

- Do you smoke or drink any alcohol?
- The doctor asked if I smoked or drank any alcohol.

- Have you had any urticaria after intravenous contrast injections?
- The doctor asked me whether I had had any urticaria after intravenous contrast injections or not.

- Are you taking any pills or medicines at the moment?
- The doctor asked me if I was taking any pills or medicines at that moment.

Wh… Questions

We use the same question word as in the *wh…* question:

- What do you mean by saying you are feeling under the weather?
- The doctor asked me what I meant by saying I was feeling under the weather.

- Why do you think you feel under the weather?
- The doctor asked me why I thought I felt under the weather.

- When do you feel under the weather?
- The doctor asked me when I felt under the weather.

- How often do you have headaches?
- The doctor asked how often I had headaches.

Reported Questions

Reported questions have the following characteristics:

- The word order is different from that of the original question. The verb follows the subject as in an ordinary statement.
- The auxiliary verb *do* is not used.
- There is no question mark.
- The verb changes in the same way as in direct speech.

Study the following examples:

- How old are you?
- The doctor asked me how old I was.

- Do you smoke?
- The doctor asked me if I smoked.

Reporting Orders and Requests

<table>
<tr><td>F O R M</td><td>

Tell (pronoun) + object (indirect) + infinitive:
- Take the pills before meals.
- The doctor told me to take the pills before meals.
- You mustn't smoke.
- The doctor told me not to smoke.
</td></tr>
</table>

Reporting Suggestions and Advice

Suggestions and advice are reported in the following forms:

- Suggestions
  - Why don't we pre-amplify the samples prior to RT-PCR?
  - The scientist suggested pre-amplifying the samples prior to RT-PCR.

- Advice
  - You should keep the tissue samples at −70 degrees Celsius.
  - The scientist advised me to keep the tissue samples at −70 degrees Celsius.

Questions

In sentences with *to be, to have* (in its auxiliary form), and modal verbs, we usually make questions by changing the word order:

- Affirmative
  - You are a scientist.
  - Interrogative: Are you a scientist?

- Negative
  - You are not a scientist.
  - Interrogative: Aren't you a scientist?

In simple present questions we use *do/does*:

- Yes, I understand the protocol.
- Do you understand the protocol?

- No, she doesn't. She takes the bus.
- Does your boss drive to work?

In simple past questions we use *did*:

- The technician arrived on time.
- Did the technician arrive on time?

If *who/what/which* is the subject of the sentence we do not use *do*:

- Dr. Di Prata phoned Dr. Smith.
- Who phoned Dr. Smith?

If *who/what/which* is the object of the sentence we use *did*:

- Dr. Smith phoned Dr. Di Prata.
- Who did Dr. Smith phone?

When we ask somebody and begin the question with *Do you know...* or *Could you tell me...*, the rest of the question maintains the affirmative sentence's word order:

- Where is the cold room?

but

- Do you know where the cold room is?
- Where is the canteen?

but

- Could you tell me where the canteen is?

Reported questions also maintain the affirmative sentence's word order:

- Dr. Wilson asked: How are you?

but

- Dr. Wilson asked me how I was.

Short answers are possible in questions where *be*, *do*, *can*, *have*, and *might* are auxiliary verbs:

- Do you smoke? Yes, I do.
- Did you smoke? No, I didn't.
- Can you walk? Yes, I can.

We also use auxiliary verbs with *so* (affirmative) and *neither* or *nor* (negative) changing the word order:

- I am feeling tired. So am I.
- I can't remember the name of the disease. Neither can I.
- Is he going to pass the exams? I think so.
- Will you be in the lab tomorrow? I guess so.

- Will you be in the lab on the weekend? I hope not.
- Has the Chairman been invited to the party? I'm afraid so.

Tag Questions

We use a positive tag question with a negative sentence and vice versa:

- The PhD student isn't feeling very well today, is she?
- You are working late at the lab, aren't you?

After *let's* the tag question is *shall we?*

- Let's read a couple of articles, shall we?

After the imperative, the tag question is *will you?*

- Turn off the laser, will you?

Infinitive/-*Ing*

Verb + -*Ing*

There are certain verbs that are usually used in the structure verb + -*ing* when followed by another verb:

- *Stop*: Please *stop talking*.
- *Finish*: I've *finished* translating the article into English.
- *Enjoy*: I *enjoy talking* to patients while I'm doing an ultrasound on them.
- *Mind*: I don't *mind being* told what to do.
- *Suggest*: Dr. Knight *suggested going* to the OT and trying to operate on the aneurysm that we couldn't stent.
- *Dislike*: She *dislikes going* out late after a long day at work.
- *Imagine*: I can't *imaging you operating*. You told me you hate blood.
- *Regret*: He *regrets having gone* two minutes before his patient had seizures.
- *Admit*: The post-doc *admitted forgetting* to switch off the mercury lamp when he was done with the microscope.
- *Consider*: Have you *considered finishing* your residence in the USA?

Other verbs that follow this structure are: *avoid, deny, involve, practice, miss, postpone*, and *risk*.

The following expressions also take -*ing*:

- *Give up*: Are you going to give *up smoking*?
- *Keep on*: She *kept on interrupting* me while I was speaking.
- *Go on*: Go *on studying*, the exam will be next month.

When we are talking about finished actions, we can also use the verb *to have*:

- The post-doc *admitted forgetting* to switch off the mercury lamp.

or

- The post-doc *admitted having forgotten* to switch off the mercury lamp.

And, with some of these verbs (*admit, deny, regret,* and *suggest*), you also can use a "that..." structure:

- The post-doc *admitted forgetting* to switch off the mercury lamp.

or

- The post-doc *admitted that he had forgotten* to switch off the mercury lamp.

Verb + Infinitive

When followed by another verb, these verbs are used with verb + infinitive structure:

- *Agree*: The patient *agreed to give up* smoking.
- *Refuse*: The patient *refused to give up* smoking.
- *Promise*: I *promised to give up* smoking.
- *Threaten*: Dr. Sommerset *threatened to close* the Pharmacology department.
- *Offer*: The unions *offered to negotiate*.
- *Decide*: Dr. Smith's research assistants *decided to leave* his research team.

Other verbs that follow this structure are: *attempt, manage, fail, plan, arrange, afford, forget, learn, dare, tend, appear, seem, pretend, need,* and *intend*.

There are two possible structures after these verbs: *want, ask, expect, help, would like,* and *would prefer*:

- Verb + infinitive: I *asked to see* Dr. Knight, the surgeon who operated on my patient.
- Verb + object + infinitive: I *asked Dr. Knight to inform* me about my patient.

There is only one possible structure after the following verbs: *tell, order, remind, warn, force, invite, enable, teach, persuade,* and *get*:

- Verb + object + infinitive: *Remind me to send* the results of the experiment to Dr. Smith tomorrow morning.

There are two possible structures after the following verbs:

- *Advise:*
  - I *wouldn't advise learning* at that oncology department.
  - I *wouldn't advise you to learn* at that oncology department.
- *Allow:*
  - They *don't allow smoking* in laboratories.
  - They *don't allow you to smoke* in laboratories.

- *Permit:*
  - They *don't permit eating* at the laboratory bench.
  - They *don't permit you to eat* at the laboratory bench.

When you use *make* and *let*, you should use the structure: verb + base form (instead of verb + infinitive):

- Blood *makes me feel* dizzy (you can't say: blood *makes me to feel* …).
- Dr. Knight *wouldn't let me process the samples*.

After the following expressions and verbs you can use either *-ing* or the infinitive: *like, hate, love, can't stand*, and *can't bear*:

- She *can't stand being* alone while she is working in the laboratory late at night.
- She *can't stand to be* alone while she is working in the laboratory late at night.

After the following verbs you can use *-ing* but not the infinitive: *dislike, enjoy*, and *mind*:

- I *enjoy being* alone (not: I *enjoy to be alone*).

Would like, a polite way of saying *I want*, is followed by the infinitive:

- *Would you like to be* the chairman of the biology division?

Begin, start, and *continue* can be followed by either *-ing* or the infinitive:

- Symptoms *began to improve* after stem cell infusion.
- Symptoms *began improving* after stem cell infusion.
- Stores supplying lab reagents cannot *continue to raise* prices.
- Stores supplying lab reagents cannot *continue raising* prices.

With some verbs, such as *remember* and *try*, the use of *-ing* and infinitive after them have different meanings:

- *Remember:*
  - *I can't remember to hang* up my lab coat (I always forget to hang up my lab coat)
  - *I can't remember hanging* up my lab coat (I'm not sure whether I hung my lab coat.
  - *I remember to send* them the cell culture (I remembered, and then sent the cultures).
  - *I remember sending* them the cell cultures (I sent them the cultures, and now I can remember doing that).
- *Try:*
  - The patient *tried to keep* her eyes open while the MR examination was going on (the patient *made an* effort to keep her eyes open during the examination).
  - If your headache persists, *try asking for* a pill (ask for the pill and *see what happens*).

Verb + Preposition + -*Ing*

If a verb comes after a preposition, that verb ends in -*ing*:

- Are you *interested in working* for our university?
- *What are the advantages of developing* new scientific techniques?
- *She's not very good at learning* languages.

You can use -*ing* with *before* and *after*:

- Decontaminate your lab coat *before laundering*.
- What did you do *after finishing* your thesis?

You can use *by* + -*ing* to explain how something happened:

- You can improve your scientific English *by reading* scientific journals.

You can use -*ing* after *without*:

- You can have a heart attack *without realizing* it.

Be careful with *to* because it can either be a part of the infinitive or a preposition:

- I'm looking forward to see you again (this is NOT correct).
- I'm looking forward to seeing you again.
- I'm looking forward to the next European symposium.

Review the following verb + preposition expressions:

- *succeed in* finding a job
- *feel like* going out tonight
- *think about* freezing your cell lines
- *dream of* being a scientist
- *disapprove of* smoking
- *look forward to* hearing from you
- *insist on* inviting me to chair the next scientific session
- *apologize for* keeping Dr. Ho waiting
- *accuse* (someone) *of* telling lies
- *suspected of* having AIDS
- *stop from* leaving the animal facility
- *thank* (someone) *for* being helpful
- *forgive* (someone) *for* not writing to me
- *warn* (someone) *against* carrying on smoking

The following are some examples of expressions + -*ing*:

- *I don't feel like* going out tonight.
- *It's no use* trying to persuade her.
- *There's no point in* waiting for him.

- *It's not worth* taking a taxi. The university is only a short walk from here.
- *It's worth* looking again at the signals on the autoradiograph film.
- *I am having difficulty* reporting that T-tube cholangiogram.
- *I am having trouble* reporting that T-tube cholangiogram.

Countable and Uncountable Nouns

Countable Nouns

Countable nouns are things we can count. We can make them plural.

Before singular countable nouns you may use *a/an*:

- You will be attended to by *a* doctor.
- Dr. Vida is looking for *an* ecologist.

Remember to use *a/an* for jobs:

- I'm *a* scientist.

Before plural countable nouns you use *some* as a general rule:

- I've read *some* good articles on stem cells lately.
- I have *some* ideas for the project.
- I had *some* difficulties finding a job.

Don't use *some* when you are talking about general things or in negative sentences:

- Generally speaking, I like biochemistry books.
- I don't have *any* ideas for the project.

You have to use *some* when you mean some, but not all:

- *Some* doctors carry a stethoscope but radiologists don't.
- I'll lend you *some* money (not all my money).

Uncountable Nouns

Uncountable nouns are things we cannot count. They have no plural.

You cannot use *a/an* before an uncountable noun; in this case you have to use *the, some, any, much, this, his*, etc. … or leave the uncountable noun alone, without the article:

- The chairman gave me an advice (NOT correct).
- The chairman gave me *some* advice.

- I saw *an* ethanol spill onto the floor (this is NOT correct because ethanol cannot be counted).
- I saw *the* ethanol spill onto the floor.

Many nouns can be used as countable or uncountable nouns. Usually there is a difference in their meaning:

- I had *many experiences* on my rotation at the Children's Hospital (countable).
- I need *experience* to become a good research assistant (uncountable).

Some nouns are uncountable in English but often countable in other languages: *advice, baggage, behavior, bread, chaos, furniture, information, luggage, news, permission, progress, scenery, traffic, travel, trouble,* and *weather.*

Articles: *A/An* and *The*

The speaker says *a/an* when it is the first time he talks about something, but once the listener knows what the speaker is talking about, he says *the:*

- This morning I performed *a* PCR on the samples. *The PCR results* were completely concordant with previous results.

We use *the* when it is clear which thing or person we mean:

- Can you turn off *the* light.
- Where is *the* biochemistry department, please?

As a general rule, we say:

- Thep olice
- The bank
- The post office
- The fire department
- Thed octor
- The hospital
- The dentist

We say: *the* sea, *the* sky, *the* ground, *the* city, and *the* country.

We don't use *the* with the names of meals:

- What did you have for lunch/breakfast/dinner?

But we use *a* when there is an adjective before a noun:

- Thank you. It was *a* delicious dinner.

We use *the* for musical instruments:

- Can you play *the* piano?

We use *the* with absolute adjectives (adjectives used as nouns). The meaning is always plural. For example:

- The rich
- The old
- The blind
- The sick
- The disabled
- The injured
- Thep oor
- The young
- The deaf
- The dead
- The unemployed
- The homeless

We use *the* with nationality words (note that nationality words always begin with a capital letter):

- *The* British, *the* Dutch, *the* Spanish.

We don't use *the* before a noun when we mean something in general:

- I love scientists (not the scientists).

With the words *school, college, prison, jail, church* we use *the* when we mean the buildings and leave the substantives alone otherwise. We say: *go to bed, go to work*, and *go home*. We don't use *the* in these cases.

We use *the* with geographical names according to the following rules:

- Continents don't use *the*:
  - Our new resident comes from Asia.
- Countries/states don't use *the*:
  - The student that rotated in Dr. Sirolli's lab came from China.
    (except for country names that include words such as Republic, Kingdom, States...; e.g., the United States of America, the United Kingdom, and The Netherlands).

As a general rule, cities don't use *the*:

- The next International Conference on Neural Transplantation and Repair will be held in Toronto.

Islands don't use *the* with individual islands but do use it with groups:

- Dr. Holmes comes from Sicily and her husband from the Canary Islands.

Lakes don't use *the*; oceans, seas, rivers and canals do use it.

- Lake Ontario is beautiful.
- *The* Panama Canal links *the* Atlantic Ocean to *the* Pacific Ocean.

We use *the* with streets, buildings, airports, universities, etc., according to the following rules:

- Streets, roads, avenues, boulevards, and squares don't use *the*:
  - The university is sited at 15th. Avenue.

- Airports don't use *the*:
  - The plane arrived at JFK airport.

- We use *the* before publicly recognized buildings: *the* White House, *the* Empire State Building, *the* Louvre museum, *the* Prado museum, *the* CN Tower.
- We use *the* before names with of: *the* Tower of London, *the* Great Wall of China.
- Universities don't use *the*: I studied at Harvard.

Word Order

The order of adjectives is discussed in the section Adjectives under the heading Adjective Order

The *verb* and the *object* of the verb normally go together:

- I studied radiology because I like *watching images* very much (*not* I like very much watching images).

We usually say the place before the time:

- She has been Chair of the Biology department at Harvard since April 2006.

We put some adverbs in the middle of the sentence:
  If the verb is one word we put the adverb before the verb:

- I performed his carotid duplex ultrasound and *also spoke* to his family.

We put the adverb after *to be*:

- You are *always* on time.

We put the adverb after the first part of a compound verb:

- Are you *definitely* attending the safety course?

In negative sentences we put *probably* before the negative:

- I *probably* won't see you at the safety course.

We also use *all* and *both* in these positions:

- Jack and Tom are *both* able to carry out a PCR.
- We *all* felt sick after the meal.

Relative Clauses

A clause is a part of a sentence. A relative clause tells us which person or thing (or what kind of person or thing) the speaker means.

A relative clause (e.g., *who is on call?*) begins with a relative pronoun (e.g., *who, that, which, whose*).

Do you know the student *who* is talking to Dr. Sirolli?

A relative clause comes after a noun phrase (e.g., the doctor, the nurse).

Most relative clauses are defining clauses and some of them are non-defining clauses.

Defining Clauses

- *The book on developmental biology (that) you lent me is very interesting.*

The relative clause is essential to the meaning of the sentence.

Commas are not used to separate the relative clause from the rest of the sentence.

That is often used instead of *who* or *which*, especially in speech.

If the relative pronoun is the object (direct object) of the clause, it can be omitted.

If the relative pronoun is the subject of the clause, it cannot be omitted.

Non-defining Clauses

- *The first bone marrow transplant in Australia, which took place at our hospital, was a complete success.*

The relative clause is not essential to the meaning of the sentence; it gives us additional information.

Commas are usually used to separate the relative clause from the rest of the sentence.

That cannot be used instead of *who* or *which*.

The relative pronoun cannot be omitted.

Relative Pronouns

Relative pronouns are used for people and for things.

- For people:
  - Subject: *who, that*
  - Object: *who, that, whom*
  - Possessive: *whose*

- For things:
  - Subject: which, that
  - Object:w hich, that
  - Possessive: whose

Who is used only for people. It can be the subject or the object of a relative clause:

- The woman *who* had only one copy of the mutation is said to have sickle cell anemia.

Which is used only for things. Like *who*, it can be the subject or object of a relative clause:

- The materials *which* are used for pronuclear microinjection of mouse zygotes are very expensive.

That is often used instead of *who* or *which*, especially in speech.

Whom is used only for people. It is grammatically correct as the object of a relative clause, but it is very formal and is not often used in spoken English. We can use *whom* instead of *who* when *who* is the object of the relative clause or when there is a preposition after the verb of the relative clause:

- The graduate student *who* I am going to the meeting with is very nice.
- The graduate student with *whom* I am going to the meeting is a very nice and intelligent person.
- Who is writing the letter?
- To whom are you writing?
- The professor *who* I saw in the Dean's Office yesterday has been suspended for having an inappropriate relationship with his student.
- The professor *whom* I saw in the Dean's Office yesterday has been suspended for having an inappropriate relationship with his student.

Whose is the possessive relative pronoun. It can be used for people and things. We cannot omit *whose*:

- Technicians *whose* wages are low should be paid more.

We can leave out *who*, *which* or *that*:

- When it is the object of a relative clause.
  - The article on the spleen that you wrote is great.
  - The article on splenic embolization you wrote is great.

- When there is a preposition. Remember that, in a relative clause, we usually put a preposition in the same place as in the main clause (after the verb):
  - The congress that we are going to next week is very expensive.
  - The congress we are going to next week is very expensive.

Prepositions in Relative Clauses

We can use a preposition in a relative clause with *who*, *which*, or *that*, or without a pronoun.

In relative clauses we put a preposition in the same place as in a main clause (after the verb). We don't usually put it before the relative pronoun. This is the normal order in informal spoken English:

- This is a problem *which* we can do very little about.
- The student (*who*) I spoke to earlier isn't here now.

In more formal or written English we can put a preposition at the beginning of a relative clause. But if we put a preposition at the beginning, we can only use *which* or *whom*. We cannot use the pronouns *that* or *who* after a preposition:

- This is a problem *about which* we can do very little.
- The student *to whom* I spoke earlier isn't here now.

Relative Clauses Without a Pronoun (Special Cases)

Infinitive Introducing a Clause

We can use the infinitive instead of a relative pronoun and a verb after:

- The first, the second, … and the next
- The only
- Superlatives

For example:
- Marie Curie was the first person *to win* two Nobel Prizes.
- Rudolf Virchow was the first *to describe* glial cells.

-Ing and -Ed Forms Introducing a Clause

We can use an -ing form instead of a relative pronoun and an active verb:

- Scientists *wanting* to train abroad should have a good level of English.

We can use an -ed form instead of a relative pronoun and a passive verb:

- The scientist *injured* in the lab was taken to the hospital.

The -ing form or the -ed form can replace a verb in a present or past tense.

Why, When, and Where

We can use *why*, *when*, and *where* in a defining relative clause.
We can leave out *why* or *when*. We can also leave out *where*, but then we must use a preposition.

We can form non-defining relative clauses with *when* and *where*:

- The clinical history, *where* everything about a patient is written, is a very important document.

We cannot leave out *when* and *where* from a non-defining clause.

Adjectives

An adjective describes (tells us something about) a noun.
In English, adjectives come before nouns (old hospital) and have the same form in both the singular and the plural (new hospital, new hospitals) and in the masculine and in the feminine.

An adjective can be used with certain verbs such as *be*, *get*, *seem*, *appear*, *look* (meaning *seem*), *feel*, *sound*, *taste* …:

- He has been *ill* since Friday, so he couldn't attend the conference.
- The patient was getting *worse*.
- The pronuclear microinjection of DNA into fertilized oocytes seemed *easy*, but it wasn't.
- Myelinated axons appear *black* when stained with Sudan Black.
- You look rather *tired*. Have you tested your RBC?
- She felt *sick*, so she stopped the renal transplant scan.
- Food in hospitals tastes *horrible*.

As you can see, in these examples there is no noun after the adjective.

Adjective Order

We have *fact adjectives* and *opinion adjectives*. Fact adjectives (*large, new, white,* ...) give us objective information about something (size, age, color, ...). Opinion adjectives (*nice, beautiful, intelligent,* ...) tell us what someone thinks of something.

In a sentence, opinion adjectives usually go before fact adjectives:

- An *intelligent* (opinion) *young* (fact) research associate visited me this morning.
- Dr. Spencer has a *nice* (opinion) *red* (fact) Porsche.

Sometimes there are two or more fact adjectives describing a noun, and generally we put them in the following order:

1. Size/length
2. Shape/width
3. Age
4. Color
5. Nationality
6. Material

For example:

- A tall young student.
- A small round lesion.
- A black latex leaded pair of gloves.
- A large new white latex leaded pair of gloves.
- An old American professor.
- A tall young Italian post-doc.
- A small square old yellow metal Geiger Counter.

Regular Comparison of Adjectives

The form used for a comparison depends upon the number of syllables in the adjective.

Adjectives of One Syllable
One-syllable adjectives (for example *fat, thin, tall*) are used with expressions of the form:

- *less ... than*(inferiority)
- *as ... as* (equality)
- *-er ... than* (superiority)

For example:

- Getting research grants is *less hard than* a few years ago.
- Eating in the hospital is *as cheap as* eating at the Medical School.
- Ultrasound examinations are difficult nowadays because people tend to be *fatter than* in the past.

Adjectives of Two Syllables

Two-syllable adjectives (for example *easy*, *dirty*, *clever*) are used with expressions of the form:

- *less … than*(inferiority)
- *as … as* (equality)
- *-er/more … than* (superiority)

We prefer *-er* for adjectives ending in *y* (*easy*, *funny*, *pretty* …) and other adjectives (such as *quiet*, *simple*, *narrow*, *clever* …). For other two-syllable adjectives we use *more*.

For example:

- The technical problem is *less simple than* you think.
- My arm is *as painful as* it was yesterday.
- The board exam was *easier than* we expected.
- His illness was *more serious than* we first suspected, as demonstrated on the high-resolution chest CT.

Adjectives of Three or More Syllables

Adjectives of three or more syllables (for example *difficult*, *expensive*, *comfortable*) are used with expressions of the form:

- *less … than*(inferiority)
- *as … as* (equality)
- *more … than* (superiority)

For example:

- Studying medicine in Spain is *less expensive than* in the States.
- The small hospital was *as comfortable* as a hotel.
- The results were *more interesting than* I had thought.

Before the comparative of adjectives you can use:

- *a (little) bit*
- *a little*
- *much*
- *a lot*
- *far*

For example:

- I am going to try something *much simpler* to solve the problem.
- The patient is *a little better* today.
- The little boy is *a bit worse* today.

Sometimes it is possible to use two comparatives together (when we want to say that something is changing continuously):

- It is becoming *more and more* difficult to find a job in the pharmaceutical industry.

We also *say twice as … as, three times as … as*:

- Going to the American Society for Neuroscience meeting *is twice as expensive as* going to the German one.

The Superlative

The form used for a superlative depends upon the number of syllables in the adjective:

Adjectives of One Syllable
One-syllable adjectives are used with expressions of the form:

- *the … -est*
- *the least*

For example:

- The number of scientists in your country is the *highest* in the world.

Adjectives of Two Syllables
Two-syllable adjectives are used with expressions of the form:

- *the … -est/I*
- *the least*

For example:

- Phosphorus-32 (32P) is one of the *commonest* radioactive isotopes used in basic research.
- Phosphorus-32 (32P) is one of the *most common* radioactive isotopes used in basic research.

Adjectives of Three or More Syllables
Adjectives of three or more syllables are used with:

- *the most*
- *the least*

For example:

- Common sense and patience are *the most important* things for a scientist.
- This is the *least difficult* brain CT I have reported in years.

Irregular Forms of Adjectives

- good   better the best
- bad   worse the worst
- far farther/further the farthest/furthest

For example:

- My ultrasound technique is *worse* now than during my first year of residence in spite of having attended several ultrasound refresher courses.

Comparatives with *The*

We use *the* + comparative to talk about a change in one thing which causes a change in something else:

- The nearer the X-ray focus the better image we have.
- The more you practice ultrasound the easier it gets.
- The higher the contrast amount the greater the risk of renal failure.

As

Two things happening at the same time or over the same period of time:

- The PhD student listened carefully *as* Dr. Fraser explained to his staff the results obtained by the two techniques was unsatisfactory.
- The accident occurred as I was leaving the laboratory.

One thing happening during another:

- The patient died *as* the CT scan was being performed.
- I had to leave the meeting just *as* the stem cell discussion was getting interesting.

Note that we use *as* only if two actions happen together. If one action follows another we don't use *as*, we use the particle *when*:

- *When* the injured scientist came to my office, I decided to call the ambulance.

Meaning *because*:

- *As* I was feeling sick, I decided to go to the doctor.

Like and *As*

Like

Like is a preposition, so it can be followed by a noun, pronoun or *-ing* form.

It means *similar to* or *the same as*. We use it when we compare things:

- Under a microscope, adipose tissue looks like a collection of bubbles.
- What does he do? He is a scientist, *like* me.

As

As + subject + verb:

- Don't change the anesthetic dose. Leave everything *as* it is.
- The tissue sample should have been treated *as* I showed you.

Meaning *what*:

- The student did *as* he was told.
- He carried out the experiment with only one sample, *as* I expected.
- *As* you know, we are sending an article to Nature Neuroscience next week.
- *As* I thought, the sample was contaminated.

As can also be a preposition, so it can be used with a noun, but it has a different meaning from *like*.

As + noun is used to say what something really is or was (especially when we talk about someone's job or how we use something):

- Before becoming a research scientist I worked *as* a research technician in a small village.

As if, *as though* are used to say how someone or something looks, sounds, feels, …, or to say how someone does something:

- The principal investigator treated me *as if* I were an undergraduate student.
- John sounds *as though* he has got a cold.

Expressions with *as*:

- *Such as*
- *As usual* (Dr. Mas was late as usual.)

So and *Such*

So and *such* make the meaning of the adjective stronger.

We use *so* with an adjective without a noun or with an adverb:

- The first-year PhD student is *so clever*.
- The animal technician injected the drug *so carefully* that the animal did not notice it.

We use *such* with an adjective with a noun:

- She is such a *clever student*.

Prepositions

At/On/In Time

We use *at* with times:

- *At* 7 o'clock
- *At* midnight
- *At* breakfast time
- *At* noon (*At* midday in British English)

We usually leave out *at* when we ask (*at*) *what time*:

- *What time* are you reporting this evening?
- *What time* are you leaving the lab tonight?

We also use *at* in these expressions:

- *At* night
- *At* the moment
- *At* the same time
- *At* the beginning of
- *At* the end of

For example:

- I don't like to work alone *at night*.
- Dr. Knight is giving a seminar *at the moment*.

We use *in* for longer periods of time:

- *In* June
- *In* summer
- *In* 1977

We also say *in the morning, in the afternoon, in the evening*:

* I'll give you the lab report *in the morning.*

We use *on* with days and dates:

* *On* October 24th
* *On* Monday
* *On* Saturday mornings
* *On* the weekend (*At* the weekend in British English)

We do not use *at/in/on* before *last* and *next*:

* I'll be in the laboratory *next* Saturday.
* They bought a new scanner *last* year.

We use *in* before a period of time (i.e., a time in the future):

* Our student went to Boston to do a rotation in Dr MacDonald's laboratory. He'll be back *in* a year.

For, During, and While

We use *for* to say to how long something takes:

* I've worked as a lab technician at this university *for* ten years.

You cannot use *during* in this way.

* It rained *for* five days (not *during* five days).

We use *during* + noun to say when something happens (not how long):

* The student fell asleep *during* the safety meeting.

We use *while* + subject + verb:

* The student fell asleep *while* he was attending the safety meeting.

By and Until

By + a time (i.e., not later than; you cannot use *until* with this meaning):

* I mailed the article on hybrid human-animal embryos today, so they should receive it *by* Tuesday.

Until can be used to say how long a situation continues:

* Let's wait *until* the patient gets better.

When you are talking about the past, you can use *by the time*:

* *By the time* they got to the hotel the congress had already started.

In/At/On

We use *in* as in the following examples:

* *In* a room
* *In* a building
* *In* a town/*in* a country (Dr. Vida works *in* Cordoba.)
* *In* the water/ocean/river
* *In* a row
* *In* the hospital

We use *at* as in the following examples:

* *At* the bus stop
* *At*t hed oor/window
* *At* the top/bottom
* *At* the airport
* *At* work
* *At* sea
* *At* an event (I saw Dr. Jules *at* the residents' party.)

We use *on* as in the following examples:

* *On* the ceiling
* *On* the floor
* *On*t he wall
* *On* a page
* *On* your nose
* *On* a farm

In or At?

* We say *in the corner of a room*, but *at the corner of a street*.
* We say *in* or *at* college/school. Use *at* when you are thinking of the college/school as a place or when you give the name of the college/school:
  - Thomas will be *in* college for three more years.
  - He studied medicine *at* Harvard Medical School.

* With buildings, you can use *in* or *at*.
* *Arrive*. We say:
  - *Arrive in* a country or town (Dr. Vida *arrived in* Boston yesterday.)
  - *Arrive at* other places (Dr. Vida *arrived at* the airport a few minutes ago.)
  - But: *arrive home* (Dr. Vida *arrived home* late after sending the article to Nature.)

Ellipsis

An ellipsis is a punctuation symbol that indicates an intentional omission of a word or a phrase from an original text. In addition, in the grammar of a sentence an ellipsis is a construction that lacks an element, which is omitted because the logic or pattern of the whole sentence makes it unnecessary. Redundant information is often omitted in conversational English. Obviously, native-English speakers use ellipsis to a greater extent than non-native-English speakers. Using ellipsis appropriately is a sign of fluency in any language. Ellipsis can be used in replies, at the beginning of a sentence, at the end of a sentence, to substitute a whole infinitive, after auxiliary verbs, and with a variety of conjunctions, pronouns and prepositions among others. Take a minute to look at the examples below.

Can you speak English? Yes, I can.
The short answer *Yes, I can*, means *Yes, I can speak English*. Both are grammatically correct, but the long answer (without ellipsis) is generally not the choice that most native-English speakers make when answering the question.

What is your name? John
The short answer *John*, means, *My name is John*.

Where are my samples? In the cold room.
The short answer *In the cold room*, means, *Your samples are in the cold room*.

Are you and John going to the Neuroscience meeting in Toronto ? We hope to.
The short answer *We hope to*, means, *Yes, we hope to go to the Neuroscience meeting in Toronto*.

Have you finished making the solutions? Yes, I have.
The short answer *Yes, I have*, means, *Yes, I have finished making the solutions*.

He worked in Dr. Smith's laboratory, and so did I. (with ellipsis)
He worked in Dr. Smith's laboratory, and I worked in Dr. Smith's laboratory too. (without ellipsis)

Which tubes are you going to use? These.
The short answer *These*, means, *I am going to use these tubes*.

UNIT III

Unit III   Usual Mistakes Made by Scientists Speaking and Writing in English

In this section we try to share with you what we have found to be some of the great hurdles in scientific English. There are many things that certainly can go wrong when one is asked to give a lecture in English or whenever one is supposed to communicate in English, and there are specific units to discuss those. This unit is by no means an exhaustive account. After reviewing English grammar usage, we think it is useful to pass our recollection of the commonest mistakes from what we have learnt from our own experience in the fascinating world of scientific English.

We have grouped these usual mistakes into four danger zones, in the hope that their classification will make them become less of a problem. The categories are the following:

1. Misnomers and false friends
2. Common grammatical mistakes
3. Common spelling mistakes
4. Common pronunciation mistakes

Misnomers and False Friends

Every tongue has its own false friends. A thorough review of false friends is beyond the scope of this manual, and we suggest that you look for those tricky names that sound similar in your language and in English but have completely different meanings.

Think, for example, about the term *graft versus host disease*. The translation of *host* has not been correct in some romance languages, and in Spanish the term *host*, which in this context means recipient, has been translated as *huésped* which means *person staying in another's house*. Many Spanish medical students and patients have problems understanding this disease because of the terminology used. Taking into account that what actually happens is that the graft reacts against the recipient, if the disease had been named *graft versus recipient disease*, the concept would probably be more precisely conveyed.

R. Ribes et al., *English for Biomedical Scientists*,
DOI: 10.1007/978-3-540-77127-2_3, © Springer-Verlag Berlin Heidelberg 2009

So from now on, identify false friends in your own language and make a list beginning with those belonging to your specialty; it is no use knowing false friends in a language different from your own.

Common Grammatical Mistakes

These are some of the most common mistakes made by scientists speaking in English:

1. The biology seminar will be held in the university library in the third floor.
   Non-native speakers often choose the wrong preposition. In general, we use "on" for a surface and "in" for an enclosed space.
   • The biology seminar will be held in the university library on the third floor.

2. You cannot go in to the radioactive room while an experiment is in progress.
   Into/in often cause a lot of confusion for non-native speakers of English.
   • You cannot go into the radioactive room while an experiment is in progress.

3. The complex binds to the 5'-end of a mRNA molecule.
   Although *a messenger ribonucleic acid…* is correct, when you use the acronym do not forget that "m" is read "em" which starts with a vowel, so the article to be used is "an" instead of "a". In this case you should write:
   • The complex binds to the 5'-end of an mRNA molecule.

4. The chairman of biology came from an university hospital.
   Although university starts with a vowel, and you may think the article which must precede it is "an" as in "an airport", the "u" is pronounced "you" which starts with a consonant, so the article to be used is "a" instead of "an". In this case you should write:
   • The chairman of biology came from a university hospital.

5. A 22-years-old man presenting …
   Many times the first sentence of the first slide of a presentation contains the first error. For those lecturers at an intermediate level, this simple mistake is so evident that they barely believe it is one of the most frequent mistakes ever made.
   It is quite obvious that the adjective *22-year-old* cannot be written in the plural and it should be written:
   • A 22-year-old man presenting …

6. There was not biopsy of the tissue.
   This is a frequent and relatively subtle mistake made by upper-intermediate speakers. If you still prefer the use of the negative form you should say:
   • There was not *any* biopsy of the tissue.
   But the affirmative form is:
   • There was no biopsy of the lesion.

7. It allows to distinguish between …
   You should use one of the following phrases:
   - It allows us to distinguish between …
   or
   - It allows the distinction between …

8. The behaviour of the labeled cells was visualized by in situ hybridisation.
   Check your paper or presentation for inconsistency in the use of American and British English.
   This example shows a sentence made up of American English words (*labeled* and *visualized*) and British English words (*behaviour* and *hybridisation*). So choose American or British spelling depending on the journal or congress you are sending your paper to.
   The sentence should read:
   - The behaviour of the labelled cells was visualised by in situ hybridisation.
   or
   - The behavior of the labeled cells was visualized by in situ hybridization

9. Please would you tell me where is the IR suite?
   Embedded questions are always troublesome. Whenever a question is embedded in another interrogative sentence its word order changes. This happens when, trying to be polite, we incorrectly change *What time is it?* to *Would you please tell me what time is it?* instead of to *Would you please tell me what time it is?*
   The direct question *where is the IR suite?* must be transformed to its embedded form as follows:
   - Please would you tell me where the IR suite is?

10. Most of the times hemangiomas …
    You can say *many times* but not *most of the times*. *Most of the time* is correct and you can use *commonly* or *frequently* as equivalent terms. Say instead:
    - Most of the time hemangiomas …

11. I look forward to hear from you.
    This a very frequent mistake at the end of formal letters such as those sent to editors. The mistake is based upon a grammatical error. *To* may be either a part of the infinitive or a preposition. In this case *to* is not a part of the infinitive of the verb *hear* but a part of the prepositional verb *look forward*; it is indeed a preposition.
    There may be irreparable consequences of making this mistake. If you are trying to have an article published in a prestigious journal you cannot make formal mistakes which can preclude the reading of your otherwise interesting article.
    So instead of *look forward to hear from you*, you should write:
    - I look forward to hearing from you.

12. Best regards.

    Although it is used in both academic and informal electronic correspondence *best regards* is a mixture of two strong English collocations: *kind regards* and *best wishes*. In our opinion instead of *best regards*, which is colloquially acceptable, you should write:
    * Kindr egards
    ors imply
    * Regards

13. A Unique metastases was seen in the liver of mice treated with the monoclonal antibodies.

    Unique and metastases are incompatible terms since the former refers to singular and the latter to plural. Therefore, the appropriate sentence should have been:
    * A unique metastasis was seen in the liver of mice treated with the monoclonal antibodies.

14. Multiple metastasis were seen in the brain.

    Multiple and metastases are incompatible terms since the former refers to plural and the latter to singular. Whenever you use a Latin term check its singular and plural forms. Metastasis is singular whereas metastases is plural so that *there are multiple metastasis* is not correct. In this case, you should write:
    * Multiple metastases were seen in the brain.

15. An European expert on stem cells chaired the session.

    Although European starts with a vowel and you may think the article which must precede it is "an" as in "an airport", the correct sentence, in this case, would be:
    * European expert on stem cells chaired the session.

16. Thel ab meeting began a hour ago.

    Although hour starts with a consonant and you may think the article which must precede it is "a" as in "a cradle", the correct sentence, in this case, would be:
    * The lab meeting began an hour ago.
    Words starting with a silent "h" are preceded by "an" as if they started with a vowel.

17. The senior technician operates on the confocal microscope for everyone in the lab.

    This sentence is not correct since the verb "to operate" carries the preposition "on" when it is used from a surgical point of view (with regard to both patients and parts of the anatomy) but not when it refers to operation of machinery or equipment. The correct sentence would have been:
    * The senior technician operates the confocal microscope for everyone in the lab.

18. Tissue was sectioned on the coronal plane into 0.5 mm-thick slices using a vibratome.
    We use "in" when talking about planes (coronal, axial, sagittal …).
    - Tissue was sectioned in the coronal plane into 0.5 mm-thick slices using a vibratome.

19. The research institute personal are very kind.
    Personal is an adjective and relates to a person. On the other hand, the word "personnel" is a noun and relates to the employees of an institution or company. The correct word is "personnel," not "personal."
    - The research institute personnel are very kind.

20. Page to the veterinarian in charge of the animal facility.
    The verb "to page" which could be related to the substantive "page" (a boy who is employed to run errands) is not a phrasal verb and does not need the preposition "to" after it. When you want the vet paged you must say:
    - Page the veterinarian in charge of the animal facility.

21. She works in the neurorradiology division.
    This is a common mistake made by Spanish and Latin American scientists. In English, neuroradiology is written with one "r":
    - She works in the neuroradiology division.

Here is another example:

He works in the neurooncology department. (incorrect).

In this case neuroncology can be written with one or two "o". If you keep both "o" you must add a hyphen between them.

- He works in the neuroncology department. (correct)
- He works in the neuro-oncology department. (correct)

Common Spelling Mistakes

Create your own list of potentially misspelled words and don't hesitate to write down your own mnemonic if it helps you.

The following is a list of commonly misspelled words (with the most common misspelling given in parentheses):

- Parallel (misspelled: paralell)
- Appearance(misspelled: apperance)

We've seen this mistake more than once in manuscripts.

- Sagittal (misspelled: saggital)

In a word with double consonants and single consonants, avoid doubling the single consonant and vice versa. Sagittal is a commonly misspelled word.

- Dura mater (misspelled: dura matter)

Etymologically "mater" means "mother" and is written with one "t". "Dura matter" is a common mistake based upon the mixing up of "dura mater" and "gray/white matter". "Matter" means substance and has nothing to do with "mater".

- Arrhythmia(misspelled: arrhytmia)

Double-check the spelling of arrhythmia and be sure that the word "rhythm" from which it is derived is embedded in it.

Review the following further pairs of words (with the misspelling given in parentheses) and, more importantly, as we said above, create your own list of "troublesome" words.

- Professor(proffesor)
- Professional (proffesional)
- Occasion (ocassion)
- Accommodate (accommodate)
- Resection (ressection)
- Gray-white matter (gray-white mater)
- Subtraction (substraction)
- Acquisition (adquisition)
- Reference(referance)
- Acquire (adquire)
- Misspell(mispell)
- Exceed (excede)
- Argument (arguement)
- A lot (allot)
- Neurogenesis (neurogenisis)
- Confocal imaging (confocol imaging)
- Acceptable (aceptable)

Common Pronunciation Mistakes

For simplicity, we have taken the liberty of using an approximate representation of the pronunciation instead of using the phonetic signs. We apologize to our linguist colleagues who may have preferred a more orthodox transcription.

Pronunciation is one of the most dreaded nightmares of English. Although there are pronunciation rules, there are so many exceptions that you must know the pronunciation of most words by ear. Therefore, firstly, read out loud as much as you can because it is the only way you will notice the unknown words with regard to pronunciation, and secondly, when you attend a course, besides concentrating on the presentation itself, focus on the way native-English-speaking scientists pronounce the words you do not know.

With regard to pronunciation, we recommend that you should:

- Not be afraid of sounding different or funny. English sounds *are* different and funny. Sometimes a non-native-speaking scientist may know how to pronounce a word correctly but is a bit ashamed of doing so, particularly in the presence of colleagues of the same nationality. Do not be ashamed of pronouncing correctly independently of the nationality of your interlocutor.
- Enjoy the effort of using a different set of muscles in the mouth. In the beginning the "English muscles" may become stiff and even hurt, but persevere, this is only a sign of hard work.
- Don't worry about having a broad or even embarrassing accent in the beginning; it doesn't matter as long as you are understood. The idea is to communicate, to say what you think or feel, and not to give a performance in speech therapy.
- Try to pronounce English words properly. As time goes by and you begin to feel relatively confident about your English, we encourage you to progressively and thoroughly study English phonetics. Bear in mind that if you keep your pronunciation as it was at the beginning you will sound like American or British people do when speaking your language with their unmistakable accent.
- Rehearse standard collocations in both conversational and scientific scenarios. Saying straightforward things such as "Do you know what I mean?" or "Would you do me a favor?" and "Where are the samples" will provide you with extremely useful fluency tools.

Having your own *subtle* national accent in English is not a serious problem as long as the presentation conveys the correct message. However, as far as pronunciation is concerned, there are several tricky words that cannot be properly named false friends and need some extra attention.

In English there are some words that are spelled differently but sound very much the same. Consider the following, for example:

- Write: make words appear on a surface such as a paper. "Write your message in the space provided."
- Right: correct, as in "the right answer"

Again, consider the following:

The English word *tear* means two different things according to how we pronounce it:

- If *tear* [tiar] is pronounced, we mean the watery secretion of the lacrimal glands which serves to moisten the conjunctiva.
- If *tear* [tear] is pronounced, we are referring to the action of wounding or injuring, especially by ripping apart as in "there is a longitudinal *tear* in the posterior horn of the internal meniscus"

Another example:

The English word *record* means two different things according to how we pronounce it:

- If *record* is pronounced with the stress on the first syllable, we mean to keep an account of, as in "Keep your medical records between you and your doctor".
- If *record* is *pronounced* with the stress on the last syllable, we mean written evidence as in "record all of your observations during your experiment in a labn otebook".

Our advice is: create a top-100 list with your day-to-day most difficult words in terms of spelling. Once you are familiar with them enlarge your list by keeping on reading out loud as many articles as you can.

We have created a list made up of some mispronounced scientific words. Since this list is absolutely arbitrary and could vary depending on your native tongue, we encourage you to create your own list.

- Parenchyma
  Parenchyma is, in principle, an easy word to pronounce. We include it in this list because we've noticed that some lecturers, particularly Italians, tend to say [pa-ren-kái-ma].

- The letter "h"
  – "Silent h": Italian and French speakers tend to skip this letter so that when they pronounce the word "enhancement" they say [en-áns-ment] instead of [en-háns-ment]. It is true that "h" can be silent but NOT always.
  – "Over-pronunciation": Spanish speakers tend to over-pronounce the letter "h".

- Disease/decease
  The pronunciation of *disease* can be funny since depending on how you pronounce the first "s" you can be saying "decease" which is what terminal diseases end in. The correct pronunciation of *disease* is "di-ssís" with a liquid "s"; if you say "di-sís" with a plain "s", as many Spanish and Latin American speakers do, every time you talk about, let's say, Alzheimer's disease, you are talking about Alzheimer's decease or Alzheimer's death.

- Hippocampus (think of *hippopotamus*)
  A lack of etymological knowledge is responsible for this tricky mistake. Many doctors worldwide say [haipo-cam-pus] as if they were talking about the hypothalamus [haipo-ta-la-mus]. Unfortunately, hippocampus has no etymological relationship to hypothalamus or hypotension. *Hippo-* means "horse" (as in *hippopotamus*) and is pronounced [hipo-cám-pus].

- Director
  Although you can say both "di-rect" and "dai-rect" only "dai-rec-tor" is correct; you cannot say "di-rec-tor"

It is beyond the scope of this manual to go over all potentially tricky words in terms of pronunciation, but we offer below a short list of more such words, and would again encourage you to create your own "personal" list.

- Medulla (me-dú-la)
- Edema (e-di-ma)
- Case report (kéis ri-pórt, NOT kéis ré-port)
- Multidetector (multi-, NOT mul-tai)
- Oblique (o-blík, NOT o-bláik)
- Femoral (fí-mo-ral)
- Jugular (jiugular)
- ...

UNIT IV

Unit IV   Writing a Manuscript

In units II and III we have given you a somewhat general introduction to scientific English grammar and usage, and to some of the usual mistakes made by non-native English-speaking biomedical scientists. In this unit, we leave introductions behind and dive in for one of the most important skills that every non-native scientist must develop: the capacity to deliver good scientific writing in English. The premise to this statement can be briefly put as follows:

1. English is not just the global language of science; it is virtually its only language.
2. Science is not really science until published (i.e. written – peer reviewed – published).
3. As a biomedical scientist you must be able to effectively write your research in English.

This chapter is not intended to be a "Guide for Authors" such as those that you can find in any journal. Even if you still do not feel very comfortable with your English skills, our main advice remains: do not write the paper first in your own language and then translate it into English; instead, do it in English directly.

Principles of Scientific Writing in English as a Foreign Language

English is a complicated language, as all our non-native readers have had the opportunity to experience. Expressing a thought in English is a bit like planning a road trip. This year my wife and I have planned a road trip for our summer holiday. We have had a particularly busy year and longed for nothing but peace and quiet. So, we chose to move away from the main roads and the busiest tourist destinations and drive down secondary roads into rural areas where we can enjoy the charm of small towns. The planning of our trip this year got me thinking about scientific writing in English.

I realized that in a different state of mood we may have chosen a trip around historical places and destinations as we did a few years back. Alternatively, we could have just focused on scenic routes and driven just for the view. For sure, there were multiple alternatives, all of them valid and possibly appropriate for a good summer vacation. But, what if rather than an enjoyable holiday we were planning a trip to quickly and effectively get from point A to point B? In this case, no doubt we would have taken nothing but the highway.

R. Ribes et al., *English for Biomedical Scientists*,
DOI: 10.1007/978-3-540-77127-2_4, © Springer-Verlag Berlin Heidelberg 2009

English language gives the speaker many more diverse alternative "routes" to explore than any road network could ever provide a driver with. But when writing science, you really have no other goal than getting from A to B as effectively and clearly as possible. The readers of scientific journals are only interested in what you did, what you found and what it means, not in any literary layers that you may be able to wrap it up with. You must be clear, you must be precise, you must keep it short, and you must be direct, like a "language highway". In a nutshell, scientific writing is to English language what the highway is to a road network.

In the following sections of this unit we will give you practical advice on how to structure your manuscript, including examples for direct, clear, concise writing. We understand well the frustration that stylistic efforts in a second language can bring on to the non-native speaker. While we encourage such efforts, you mustn't forget that your real target is no more than putting together a well-organized manuscript that clearly portrays your quality results. Even if the style isn't perfect the copyeditors of the journal will be able to make necessary stylistic corrections. However, if the message of your research is not clearly presented, if it does not include clear information about your data, there is nothing that the editing process will be able to do to fix it. Your best model to write a manuscript about your topic for a particular journal is another manuscript in the same journal. Use effective imitation as a source to get right the structure of your paper, the layout of paragraphs, or the level of detail, to mention a few aspects. In case of doubt, always keep your wording and sentence structure simple. Choose the shortest, most direct version that works. Finally, if at all feasible, have a colleague with a good command of written scientific English to review your manuscript before submission.

Preliminary Work

When you have a subject that you want to report, first of all you need to look up references. You can refer to the *Index Medicus* (http://www.ncbi.nlm.nih. gov/entrez/query.fcgi?db=PubMed) to search for articles. Once you have found them, read them thoroughly and underline those sentences or paragraphs that you think you might quote in your article.

As mentioned earlier, our advice is not to write the paper in your own language and then translate it into English; instead, write in English directly. In order to do so, pick up, either out of these references, or out of the journal in which you want your work to be published, the article that you find closest to the type of study that you want to report.

Although you must follow the instructions of the journal to which you want to send the paper, here we use a standard form that may be adequate for most of them. In each section, we give you a few examples just to show how you can get them from other articles.

Article Header

Title

The title of the article should be concise but informative. Put a lot of thought into the title of your article.

Abstract

An abstract of 150–250 words (it depends on the journal) must be submitted with each manuscript. Remember that an abstract is a synopsis, *not* an introduction to the article.

The abstract should answer the question: "What should readers know after reading this article."

Most journals require that the abstract is divided into four paragraphs with the following headings.

Objective

To state the purposes of the study or investigation, the hypothesis being tested, or the procedure being evaluated.

Notice that very often you may construct the sentence beginning with an infinitive tense:

- *To evaluate* the effects of interferons (IFNs) in experimental autoimmune encephalomyelitis (EAE) mice.
- *To present* our experience with Affymetrix Gene Chips.
- *To study* the role of Sox10 in early neural crest development.
- *To assess* the effects of botulinum toxin in the treatment of cerebral palsy.
- *To compare* the image acquisition time for digital versus film-screen imaging for screening mammography in a hard-copy interpretation environment.
- *To determine* the origin of oligodendrocytes in the developing mouse telencephalon using a Cre-lox genetic fate mapping approach.
- *To develop* an efficient and fully unsupervised method to quantitatively assess myocardial contraction from 4D-tagged MR sequences.
- *To investigate* the role of p53 on the induction of apoptosis and cell cycle arrest in zebrafish.
- *To ascertain* recent trends in imaging workload among the various medical specialties.
- *To describe* the clinical and biological characteristics of Krabbe's disease in rhesus macaques.

- *To characterize* the expression pattern of PLP in jimpy mice.
- *To assess* the usefulness of the Mouse Information and Classification Entity (MICE) program to track and monitor research animals in large vivaria.
- *To examine* the molecular mechanisms that control floor plate and notochord formation in mice.
- *To establish ..., To perform ..., To study ..., To design ..., To analyze ..., To test ..., To define ..., To illustrate ...*

You can also begin with: "The aim/purpose/objective/goal of this study was to ...."

- *The aim of this study was to* determine the distribution of Shh in normal spinal cords using immunohistochemical methods.
- *The purpose of this study was to* determine the safety and effectiveness of the MMR jab in children.
- *The goal of this investigation was to* determine if overexpression of PDGF-A increased the number of oligodendrocyte progenitor cells in the mouse spinal cord.
- *The objective of this study was to* determine whether estrogen has direct effects on adipocyted evelopment.

You may give some background and then state what you have done.

- *Autoimmune pancreatitis is a new clinical entity which frequently mimics pancreatic carcinoma, resulting in unnecessary radical surgery of the pancreas. The purpose of this study was to describe radiologic findings of autoimmune pancreatitis.*
- *Myocardial fibrosis is known to occur in patients with hypertrophic cardiomyopathy (HCM) and to be associated with myocardial dysfunction. This study was designed to clarify the relation between myocardial fibrosis demonstrated by gadolinium-enhanced magnetic resonance imaging (Gd-MRI) and procollagen peptides or cytokines.*
- *It appears that oligodendrocytes (OLs) do not arise exclusively from the ventral neural tube. Both halves of the neural tube give rise to oligodendrocyte precursor cells (OLPs). It is well known that Shh is required for the specification of OLs in the ventral neural tube, because disruption of Shh signaling prevents OLPs from being generated in this region. However, Shh has never been detected in the dorsal region of the neural tube. This would suggest that dorsally-derived OLPs are generated using a different signaling pathway. The purpose of this study was to determine the extracellular signals involved in the specification of OLPs in the dorsal neural tube.*
- *.... We hypothesized that ...*
- *.... We compared ...*
- *.... We investigated ...*

Materials and Methods

Briefly state what was done and what materials were used, including the number of subjects. Also include the methods used to assess the data and to control bias.

- N *animals with ... were included.*
- N *animals with ... were excluded.*
- N *animals known to have/suspected of having ...*
- *... was performed in* N *animals with ...*
- N *animals underwent ...*
- *Quantitative/Qualitative analyses were performed by ...*
- *Patients were followed clinically for ... months/years.*
- *We examined the effects of iodinated IV contrast on blood pressure, heart rate and renal function in 14 healthy young monkeys.*

Results

Provide the findings of the study, including indicators of statistical significance. Include actual numbers, as well as percentages.

- *After 12 days culture, specific HLA tetramer binding CTL expanded up to 75% of CD8+T cells. Phenotypic analysis showed that the antigen-specific CTL were skewed towards a CCR7-/CD45RA effector memory phenotype. To study the origin of antigen-specificTem, CCR7/CD45RA CD8+ subpopulations (T_N, T_{CM}, T_{EM} and T_{TE}) were sorted and stimulated separately with peptide-pulsed DC. This demonstrated that the expansion of antigen-specific cells took place predominantly in the Tcm and Tem compartments and that the phenotype converted from Tcm to Tem. Functional analysis showed efficient cytotoxic target killing and expression of perforin, granzyme and IFN. Further analysis for CD27/28 showed that the homogenous Tem population could be further dissected into different maturation stages where CD27 expression correlated inversely with the level of IFN and perforin expression, though the majority of cells were double positive for CD27 and CD28, suggesting an early differentiation phenotype.*
- *Levels of CD25hiCD4+ Tregs were 2.35% of total CD4+ T cells +/-.42 in our patient cohort. CD25hiCD4+ levels correlated with FOXP3 expression (r=.484; p=.0001) and with TGFβ production (r=.911; p<.0001), in keeping with a true regulatory phenotype. At a median follow-up of 3 years, patients with high Tregs levels had a reduced overall survival (OS; 13% vs 52%; P=.001) and disease free survival (DFS; 13% vs 26%; P=.033) compared to patients with lower Tregs levels. Higher CD25hiCD4+ Tregs levels, however, did associate with an increased risk of relapse (80% vs 47%; P=.001), suggesting an effect of Tregs on GVT responses in this population.*

Conclusion

Summarize in one or two sentences the conclusion(s) made on the basis of the findings. Your conclusion should emphasize new and important aspects of the study or observations.

- *MO7e-G cells provide a powerful system where to dissect the molecular basis of the synergy between SCF and GCSF.*

- *Contrast enhancement characteristics of breast cancer are significantly affected by contrast injection rate. It is critical to incorporate contrast injection rate into pharmacokinetic modeling for accurate characterization of breast cancer.*
- *Our results demonstrate that the CD45RA antigen should not be used alone to define naïve CD4$^+$ T-cells when monitoring T-cell reconstitution in T-cell replete HCT recipients.*
- *US is moderately accurate in the diagnosis of substantial fatty atrophy of the supraspinatus or infraspinatus muscles.*
- *Overall, we show that preserved immune function and adequate gene-transfer are not incompatible goals for protocols of retroviral transduction of T-lymphocytes based on polyclonal expansion.*
- *The study data demonstrate ..., Preliminary findings indicate ..., Results suggest ...*

Keywords

Below the abstract you should provide, and identify as such, three to ten keywords or short phrases that will assist indexers in cross-indexing the article and may be published with the abstract. The terms used should be from the Medical Subject Headings list of the Index Medicus (http://www.nlm.nih.gov/mesh/meshhome.html).

Main Text

The text of observational and experimental articles is usually (but not necessarily) divided into sections with the headings *Introduction, Materials and Methods, Results,* and *Discussion.* Long articles may need subheadings within some sections (especially the Results and Discussion sections) to clarify their content. Other types of articles, such as Case Reports, Reviews, and Editorials, are likely to need other formats. You should consult individual journals for further guidance.

Avoid using abbreviations. When used, abbreviations should be spelled out the first time a term is given in the text, for example *magnetic resonance imaging (MRI).*

Introduction

The text should begin with an Introduction that conveys the nature and purpose of the work, and quotes the relevant literature. Give only strictly pertinent background information necessary for understanding why the topic is important and references that inform the reader as to why you undertook your study. Do not review the literature extensively. The final paragraph should clearly state the hypothesis or purpose of your study. Brevity and focus are important.

Materials and Methods

Details of clinical and technical procedures should follow the Introduction.

Describe your selection of the observational or experimental subjects (patients or laboratory animals, including controls) clearly. Identify the age, sex, and other important characteristics of the subjects. Because the relevance of such variables as age, sex, and ethnicity to the object of research is not always clear, authors should explicitly justify them when they are included in a study report. The guiding principle should be clarity about how and why a study was done in a particular way. For example, authors should explain why only subjects of certain ages were included or why women were excluded. You should avoid terms such as "race," which lack precise biological meaning, and use alternative concepts such as "ethnicity" or "ethnic group" instead. You should also specify carefully what the descriptors mean, and say exactly how the data were collected (for example, what terms were used in survey forms, whether the data were self-reported or assigned by others, etc.).

- *Our study population was selected from …*
- *N animals underwent …*
- *N consecutive animals …*
- *N animals with proven …*
- *Patients were followed clinically …*
- *N animals with … were examined before and during …*
- *N patients with known or suspected … were prospectively enrolled in this study.*
- *More than N animals presenting with … were examined with … over a period of N months.*
- *N patients were prospectively enrolled between … (date) and … (date).*
- *N patients (N men, N women; age range N–N years; mean N.N years).*
- *In total, 140 patients, aged 30–50 years (mean 40 years), all with severe acute pancreatitis fulfilling Ramson criteria, were included in the study.*
- *Patients undergoing elective coronary arteriography for evaluation of chest pain were considered eligible if …*

Identify the methods, instrumentation (trade names and manufacturer's name and location in parentheses), and procedures in sufficient detail to allow other workers to reproduce your study. Identify precisely all drugs and chemicals used, including generic name(s), dose(s), and route(s) of administration.

- *DNA template was labeled with^{32}P-dCTP using the Rediprime^{TM}II Random Prime Labelling System (Amersham Pharmacia Biotech).*
- *Pronuclear microinjection was performed under a microscope containing a working-distance condenser (Leica, Germany).*
- *Mice were purchased from a commercial breeding farm (Charles River Laboratories, UK).*
- *Automatic high-speed core biopsy equipment (Biopty instrument and Biopty-Cut needles; Bard Urological, Covington, Ga.) was used.*

- *Donor female C57BL6xCBA F1 hybrid mice (4–5 weeks of age) were superovulated with an intraperitoneal injection of 5 i.u. serum gonadotrophin (Folligon, Intervet), followed 45 hours later by 5 i.u. human chorionic gonadotropin (Chorulon®, Inervet). Gonadotropins were diluted in 0.9% sodium chloride (NaCl Injection B.P., Antigen Pharmaceuticals).*
- *Females that have been plugged by a vasectomized male were anaesthetized with a solution containing 25% of fentanyl citrate/fluanisone (Hynorm, VetaPharma Ltd.) and 25% of midazolam (Hypnovel, Roche). The induction dose was administered intraperitoneally at a dose of 5 µl/g body weight.*
- *Prehybridization was carried out in sealed roller bottles in a hybridization rotisserie oven (Hybaid Maxi-14, USA) for at least 1 hour using 100 µg/ml denatured sheared salmon sperm DNA in MIB buffer (0.225 M NaCl, 15 mM NaH2PO4, 1.5 mM EDTA, 10% PEG 8000, 7% SDS).*
- *Absolute CD4⁺ cell counts were determined using TruCOUNT technology (Becton Dickinson, UK) according to the manufacturer's instructions.*
- *Sections were incubated overnight at 4°C with GFP antibody (1:8000, Abcam, Cambridge, UK)) or Sox10 antibody (1:2000; gift from Sofia Wilson, Harvard Medical School, Boston, MA) in PBS containing 1% FCS.*

It is essential that you state the manner by which studies were evaluated: independent readings, consensus readings, blinded or unblinded to other information, time sequencing between readings of several studies of the same patient or animal to eliminate recall bias, and random ordering of studies. It should be clear as to the retrospective or prospective nature of your study.

- *Entry/inclusion criteria included …*
- *These criteria had to be met: …*
- *Patients with … were not included.*
- *Further investigations, including … and …, were also performed.*
- *We prospectively studied N patients with …*
- *The reviews were not blinded to the presence of …*
- *The following patient inclusion criteria were used: age between 16 and 50 years and closed epiphyses, ACL injury of one knee that required surgical replacement with a bone-to-patellar tendon-to-bone autograft, and signed informed consent with agreement to attend follow-up visits. The following exclusion criteria were used: additional ligament laxities with a grade higher than 2 (according to the European classification of frontal laxity) in the affected knee, …*
- *Two skeletal radiologists (O.J., C.V.) in consensus studied the following parameters on successive MR images …*
- *Both the interventional cardiologists and echocardiographers who performed the study and evaluated the results were blinded to drug administration.*
- *Histologic samples were evaluated in a blinded manner by one of the authors and an outside expert in rodent liver pathology.*

Give references to established methods, including statistical methods that have been published but are not well known; describe new or substantially modified methods, give reasons for using these techniques, and evaluate their limitations.

Identify precisely all drugs and chemicals used, including generic name(s), dose(s), and route(s) of administration. Do not use a drug's trade name unless it is directly relevant.

- *The imaging protocol included ...*
- *Cytokine-capture assay was performed following the manufacturer's instructions.*
- *To assess objectively the severity of acute pancreatitis, all patients were scored using (10).*
- *The stereotactic device used for breast biopsy has been described elsewhere (12); it consists of a ...*
- *RT-PCR was carried out as previously described (2).*

Statistics

Describe statistical methods with enough detail to enable a knowledgeable reader with access to the original data to verify the reported results. Put a general description of methods in the Methods section. When data are summarized in the Results section, specify the statistical methods used to analyze them:

- *The statistical significance of differences was calculated with Fisher's exact test.*
- *The probability of ... was calculated using the Kaplan-Meier method.*
- *To test for statistical significance, ...*
- *Statistical analyses were performed with ... and ... tests.*
- *The levels of significance are indicated by P values.*
- *Interobserver agreement was quantified by using k statistics.*
- *All P values of less than 0.05 were considered to indicate statistical significance.*
- *Univariate and multivariate Cox proportional hazards regression models were used.*
- *The v^2-test was used for group comparison. Descriptive values of variables are expressed as means and percentages.*
- *We adjusted RRs for age (5-year categories) and used the Mantel extension test to test for linear trends. To adjust for other risk factors, we used multiple logistic regression.*

Give details about randomization:

- *They were selected consecutively by one physician between February 1999 and June 2000.*
- *This study was conducted prospectively during a period of 30 months from March 1998 to August 2000. We enrolled 29 consecutive patients who had ...*

Specify any general-use computer programs used:

- *All statistical analyses were performed with SAS software (SAS Institute, Cary, N.C.).*
- *The statistical analyses were performed using SPSS for Windows, release 8.0 (SPSS, Chicago, Ill.).*
- *Stained sections were observed under a Leica TCS SP confocal microscope using Leica Confocal Software. Figures were prepared using Adobe Photoshop 6.0 software.*

- *Images were captured digitally on a Dell computer by using the SimplePCI imaging software.*
- *The sequences obtained in the study were analysed using the Sequence Analysis software package by Genetic Computers Inc.*
- *Sequences were compared with those in the NCBI database using NCBI Blast program.*

Results

Present your results in a logical sequence in the text, along with tables, and illustrations. Do not repeat in the text all the data in the tables or illustrations; emphasize or summarize only important observations. Avoid nontechnical uses of technical terms in statistics, such as "random" (which implies a randomizing device), "normal," "significant," "correlations," and "sample." Define statistical terms, abbreviations, and most symbols:

- *Statistically significant differences were shown for both X and X.*
- *Significant correlation was found between X and X.*
- *Results are expressed as means±SD.*
- *All the abnormalities in our patient population were identified on the prospective clinical interpretation.*
- *The abnormalities were correctly characterized in 14 patients and incorrectly in …*
- *The preoperative and operative characteristics of these patients are listed in Table 1.*
- *The results of the US-guided core-needle pleural biopsies are shown in Table 1.*
- *The clinical findings are summarized in Table 1.*

Report any complication:

- *Two minor complications were encountered. After the second procedure, one patient had a slight hemoptysis that did not require treatment, and one patient had local chest pain for about 1 hour after a puncture in the supraclavicular region. Pneumothorax was never encountered.*
- *Among the 11,101 patients, there were 373 in-hospital deaths (3.4%), 204 intraoperative/postoperative CVAs (1.8%), 353 patients with postoperative bleeding events (3.2%), and 142 patients with sternal wound infections (1.3%).*

Give numbers of observations. Report losses to observation (such as dropouts from a clinical trial):

- *The final study cohort consisted of …*
- *Of the 961 patients included in this study, 69 were reported to have died (including 3 deaths identified through the NDI), and 789 patients were interviewed (Figure 1). For 81 surviving patients, information was obtained from another source. Twenty-two patients (2.3%) could not be contacted and were not included in the analyses because information on nonfatal events was not available.*

Discussion

Within this section, use ample subheadings. Emphasize the new and important aspects of the study and the conclusions that follow from them. Do not repeat in detail data or other material given in the Introduction or the Results sections. Include in the Discussion section the implications of the findings and their limitations, including implications for future research. Relate the observations to other relevant studies.

Link the conclusions with the goals of the study, but avoid unqualified statements and conclusions not completely supported by the data. In particular, avoid making statements on economic benefits and costs unless the report includes economic data and analyses. Avoid claiming priority and alluding to work that has not been completed. State new hypotheses when warranted, but clearly label them as such. Recommendations, when appropriate, may be included.

- *This study demonstrates that ...*
- *This study highlights ...*
- *Another finding of our study is ...*
- *This work has clearly shown another important ...*
- *One limitation of our study was ...*
- *Other methodological limitations of this study ...*
- *Our results support ...*
- *Our data support ...*
- *Our results show ...*
- *Further research is needed to elucidate ...*
- *However, the limited case number warrants a more comprehensive study to confirm these findings and to assess the comparative predictive value of relative lung volume versus LHR.*
- *Some follow-up is probably appropriate for these patients.*
- *However, we cannot exclude the possibility that ...*
- *Our results are inconsistent with recent studies that ...*
- *Further research is needed to determine the factors associated with multiple sclerosis (MS) relapse.*
- *The data also raise new questions ...*
- *It will be interesting to determine whether ...*

Acknowledgments

List all contributors who do not meet the criteria for authorship, such as a person who provided purely technical help, writing assistance, or a department chair who provided only general support. Financial and material support should also be acknowledged.

People who have contributed materially to the paper but whose contributions do not justify authorship may be listed under a heading such as "clinical investigators" or "participating investigators," and their function or contribution should be described: for example, "served as scientific advisors," "critically reviewed the study proposal," "collected data," or "provided and cared for study patients."

Because readers may infer their endorsement of the data and conclusions, everybody must have given written permission to be acknowledged.

- *The authors express their gratitude to … for their excellent technical support.*
- *The authors thank Wei J. Chen, MD, ScD, Institute of Epidemiology, College of Public Health, National Taiwan University, Taipei, for the analysis of the statistics and his help in the evaluation of the data. The authors also thank Pan C. Yang, MD, PhD, Department of Internal Medicine, and Keh S. Tsai, MD, PhD, Department of Laboratory Medicine, National Taiwan University, Medical College and Hospital, Taipei, for the inspiration and discussion of the research idea of this study. We also thank Ling C. Shen for her assistance in preparing the manuscript.*
- *We thank Drs. Sirolli and Frade for insightful discussions and comments on this manuscript.*
- *We thank Rocco Fontana for antibodies against PLP and MBP.*
- *We are grateful to Sophia Wilson for expert help in pronuclear microinjections.*

References

References can be numbered consecutively in the order in which they are first mentioned in the text or listed alphabetically by author's last name. Identify references in text, tables, and legends by Arabic numerals in parentheses (some journals require superscript Arabic numbers). References cited only in tables or figure legends should be numbered in accordance with the sequence established by the first citation in the text of the particular table or figure.

- *Clinically, resting thallium-201 (^{201}Tl) single photon emission computed tomography (SPECT) has been widely used to evaluate myocardial viability in patients with chronic coronary arterial disease and acute myocardial infarction (8–16).*
- *Lymphoma is currently the most frequent indication for performing an HSCT in Europe. In particular, the percentage of allogeneic HSCT for lymphoma has markedly increased over the recent years due to the introduction of reduced-intensity conditioning allogeneic HSCT.[17,18]*

Use the style of the examples below, which are based on the formats used by the NLM in *Index Medicus*. The titles of journals should be abbreviated according to the style used in *Index Medicus*. Consult the *List of Journals Indexed in Index Medicus*, published annually as a separate publication by the library and as a list in the January issue of *Index Medicus*. The list can also be obtained through the library's website (http://www.nlm.nih.gov).

Avoid using abstracts as references. References to papers accepted but not yet published should be designated as "in press" or "forthcoming"; authors should obtain written permission to cite such papers as well as verification that they have been accepted for publication. Information from articles submitted but not accepted should be cited in the text as "unpublished observations" with written permission from the source.

Avoid citing a "personal communication" unless it provides essential information not available from a public source, in which case the name of the person and date of communication should be cited in parentheses in the text. For scientific articles, authors should obtain written permission and confirmation of accuracy from the source of a personal communication.

The references must be verified by the author(s) against the original documents.

The Uniform Requirements style (the Vancouver style) is based largely on an ANSI standard style adapted by the NLM for its databases. Notes have been added where Vancouver style differs from the style now used by NLM.

Articles in Journals

Standard Journal Article

List the first six authors followed by et al. (*Note*: NLM now lists up through 25 authors; if there are more than 25 authors, NLM lists the first 24, then the last author, then et al.)

Theodorou SJ, Theodorou DJ, Schweitzer ME, Kakitsubata Y, Resnick D. Magnetic resonance imaging of para-acetabular insufficiency fractures in patients with malignancy. Clin Radiol 2006 Feb;61(2):181–190.

As an option, if a journal carries continuous pagination throughout a volume, the month and issue number may be omitted. (*Note*: for consistency, the option is used throughout the examples in Uniform Requirements. NLM does not use the option.)

Theodorou SJ, Theodorou DJ, Schweitzer ME, Kakitsubata Y, Resnick D. Magnetic resonance imaging of para-acetabular insufficiency fractures in patients with malignancy. Clin Radiol 2006;61:181–190.

Organization as Author

The Evidence-based Radiology Working Group. Evidence-based radiology: a new approach to the practice of radiology. Radiology 2001;220:566–575.

No Author Given

Cancer in South Africa [editorial]. S Afr Med J 1994;84:15.

Article Not In English

(Note: NLM translates the title to English, encloses the translation in square brackets, and adds an abbreviated language designator.)

Zangos S, Mack MG, Straub R, et al. [Transarterial chemoembolization (TACE) of liver metastases: a palliative therapeutic approach]. Radiologie 2001: 41(1):84–90. German

Volume with Supplement

Shen HM, Zhang QF. Risk assessment of nickel carcinogenicity and occupational lung cancer. Environ Health Perspect 1994;102 Suppl 1:275–82.

Issue with Supplement

Payne DK, Sullivan MD, Massie MJ. Women's psychological reactions to breast cancer. Semin Oncol 1996; 23(1 Suppl 2):89–97.

Hamm B, Staks T, Taupitz M. SHU 555A: a new superparamagnetic iron oxide contrast agent for magnetic resonance imaging. Invest Radiol 1994; 29(Suppl 2): S87–S89.

Volume with Part

Ozben T, Nacitarhan S, Tuncer N. Plasma and urine sialic acid in non-insulin dependent diabetes mellitus. Ann Clin Biochem 1995; 32(Pt 3):303–6.

Issue with Part

Poole GH, Mills SM. One hundred consecutive cases of flap lacerations of the leg in ageing patients. N Z Med J 1994; 107(986 Pt 1):377–8.

Issue with No Volume

Turan I, Wredmark T, Fellander-Tsai L. Arthroscopic ankle arthrodesis in rheumatoid arthritis. Clin Orthop 1995; (320):110–4.

No Issue or Volume

Browell DA, Lennard TW. Immunologic status of the cancer patient and the effects of blood transfusion on antitumor responses. Curr Opin Gen Surg 1993: 325–33.

Pages in Roman Numerals

Fisher GA, Sikic BI. Drug resistance in clinical oncology and hematology. Introduction. Hematol Oncol Clin North Am 1995 Apr; 9(2): xi–xii.

Type of Article Indicated as Needed

Enzensberger W, Fischer PA. Metronome in Parkinson's disease [letter]. Lancet 1996; 347:1337.

Clement J, De Bock R. Hematological complications of hantavirus nephropathy (HVN) [abstract]. Kidney Int 1992;42:1285.

Article Containing Retraction

Garey CE, Schwarzman AL, Rise ML, Seyfried TN. Ceruloplasmin gene defect associated with epilepsy in EL mice [retraction of Garey CE, Schwarzman AL, Rise ML, Seyfried TN. In: Nat Genet 1994;6:426–31]. Nat Genet 1995;11:104.

Article Retracted

Liou GI, Wang M, Matragoon S. Precocious IRBP gene expression during mouse development [retracted in Invest Ophthalmol Vis Sci 1994;35:3127]. Invest Ophthalmol Vis Sci 1994;35:1083–8.

Article with Published Erratum

Hamlin JA, Kahn AM. Herniography in symptomatic patients following inguinal hernia repair [published erratum appears in West J Med 1995;162:278]. West J Med 1995;162:28–31.

Books and Other Monographs

Personal Author(s)

Helms CA. Fundamentals of skeletal radiology. 1st ed. Philadelphia: W.B. Saunders Company; 1992.

(Note: Previous Vancouver style incorrectly had a comma rather than a semicolon between the publisher and the date.)

Editor(s), Compiler(s) as Author

Rumack CM, Wilson SR, Charboneau JW, editors. Diagnostic ultrasound. St Louis: Mosby-Year Book; 1998.

Organization as Author and Publisher

Institute of Medicine (US). Looking at the future of the Medicaid program. Washington: The Institute; 1992.

Chapter in a Book

Levine MS. Benign tumors of the esophagus. In: Gore RM, Levine MS, editors. Textbook of gastrointestinal radiology. 2nd ed. Philadelphia, Pa: Saunders; 2000. pp. 387–402.

(Note: Previous Vancouver style had a colon rather than a p before pagination.)

Conference Proceedings

Kimura J, Shibasaki H, editors. Recent advances in clinical neurophysiology. Proceedings of the 10th International Congress of EMG and Clinical Neurophysiology; 1995 Oct 15–19; Kyoto, Japan. Amsterdam: Elsevier; 1996.

Conference Paper

Bengtsson S, Solheim BG. Enforcement of data protection, privacy and security in medical informatics. In: Lun KC, Degoulet P, Piemme TE, Rien?hoff O, editors. MEDINFO 92. Proceedings of the 7th World Congress on Medical Informatics; 1992 Sep 6–10; Geneva, Switzerland. Amsterdam: North-Holland; 1992. pp. 1561–5.

Scientific or Technical Report

Issued by funding/sponsoring agency:
Smith P, Golladay K. Payment for durable medical equipment billed during skilled nursing facility stays. Final report. Dallas (TX): Dept. of Health and Human Services (US), Office of Evaluation and Inspections; 1994 Oct. Report No.: HHSIGOEI69200860.

Issued by performing agency:
Field MJ, Tranquada RE, Feasley JC, editors. Health services research: work force and educational issues. Washington: National Academy Press; 1995. Contract No.: AHCPR282942008. Sponsored by the Agency for Health Care Policy and Research.

Dissertation

Kaplan SJ. Post-hospital home health care: the elderly's access and utilization [dissertation]. St. Louis (MO): Washington Univ.; 1995.

Patent

Larsen CE, Trip R, Johnson CR, inventors; Novoste Corporation, assignee. Methods for procedures related to the electrophysiology of the heart. US patent 5,529,067. 1995 Jun 25.

Other Published Material

Newspaper Article

Lee G. Hospitalizations tied to ozone pollution: study estimates 50,000 admissions annually. The Washington Post 1996 Jun 21; Sect. A:3 (col. 5).

Audiovisual Material

HIV+/AIDS: the facts and the future [videocassette]. St. Louis (MO): Mosby Year-Book; 1995.

Dictionary and Similar References

Stedman's medical dictionary. 26th ed. Baltimore: Williams & Wilkins; 1995. Apraxia; pp. 119–20.

Unpublished Material

In Press

(Note: NLM prefers "forthcoming" because not all items will be printed.)

Assessment of chest pain in the emergency room: What is the role of multidetector CT? Eur J Radiol. In press 2006.

Electronic Material

Journal Article in Electronic Format

Morse SS. Factors in the emergence of infectious diseases. Emerg Infect Dis [serial online] 1995 Jan-Mar [cited 1996 Jun 5]; 1(1):[24 screens]. Available from: URL: http://www.cdc.gov/ncidod/EID/eid.htm

Monograph in Electronic Format

CDI, clinical dermatology illustrated [monograph on CD-ROM]. Reeves JRT, Maibach H. CMEA Multimedia Group, producers. 2nd ed. Version 2.0. San Diego: CMEA; 1995.

Computer File

Hemodynamics III: the ups and downs of hemodynamics [computer program]. Version 2.2. Orlando (FL): Computerized Educational Systems; 1993.

Additional Material

Tables

All tabulated data identified as tables should be given a table number and a descriptive caption. Take care that each table is cited in numerical sequence in the text.

The presentation of data and information given in the table headings should not duplicate information already given in the text. Explain in footnotes all non-standard abbreviations used in the table.

If you need to use any table or figure from another journal, make sure you ask for permission and put a note such as:

Adapted, with permission, from reference 5.

Figures

Figures should be numbered consecutively in the order in which they are first cited in the text. Follow the "pattern" of similar illustrations of your references.

- *Figure 1. Northern blot analysis shows ...*

- *Figure 2. Cryosection from the ventral columns of a cervical spinal cord shows ...*

- *Figure 3. Selective renal arteriogram shows ...*

- *Figure 4. Photograph of a fresh-cut specimen shows ...*

- *Figure 5. Photomicrograph (original magnification, ×10; hematoxylin-eosin stain) of ...*

- *Figure 6. Histological risk associated with the outcome of liver GVHD.*

- *Figure 7. Typical metastatic compression fracture in a 65-year-old man (**a**) 1-weighted MR image (400/11) shows ...*

- *Figure 6. Nasal-type extranodal NK/T-cell lymphoma involving the nasal cavity in a 42-year-old woman. Photomicrograph (original magnification, ×400; hematoxylin-eosin [H-E] stain) of a nasal mucosal biopsy specimen shows intense infiltration of atypical lymphoid cells into the vascular intima and subintima (arrow). This is a typical appearance of angiocentric invasion in which the vascular lumen (V) is nearly obstructed.*

- *Figure 7. AFX with distortion of histopathologic architecture as a consequence of intratumoral ...*

- *Figure 8. Southern blot analysis of PAC clones confirms the presence of the Sox10 gene. Clones were digested with EcoRI and hybridized to a 3'-Sox10-UTR cDNA probe. The expected band size is 5 kb.*

Final Tips

Before you submit your article for publication check its spelling, and go over your article for words you might have omitted or typed twice, as well as words you may have misused such as using "there" instead of "their." Do not send an article with spelling or dosage errors or other medical inaccuracies. And do not expect the spell-check function on your computer to catch all your spelling mistakes.

Be accurate. Check and double-check your facts and reference citations. Even after you feel the article is finished leave it for a day or two and then go back to it. The changes you make to your article after seeing it in a new light will often be the difference between a good article and a great article.

Once you believe everything is correct, give the draft to your English teacher for a final informal editing. Do not send your first (or even second) draft to the publisher!

Do not forget to read and follow carefully the specific "Instructions for authors" of the journal in which you want your work to be published.

UNIT V

Unit V   Writing Scientific Correspondence

This unit is made up of several examples of letters sent to editors of scientific journals. Our intention is to provide you with useful tools to communicate with journal editors and reviewers in a formal manner. It is our understanding that letters to editors have quite an important, and many times overlooked, role in the fate of scientific manuscripts.

Although we are not going to focus on letters from editors since they are, generally speaking, easy to understand, these letters can be divided into acceptance "under certain conditions" letters, acceptance letters, and rejection letters.

- Acceptance "under certain conditions" letters. These letters are relatively common, and usually mean some level of work since the paper must be re-written.
- Acceptance letters. Congratulations! Your paper has finally been accepted and no corrections have to be made. These letters are, unfortunately, relatively uncommon, and quite easy to read. Besides, they do not need to be replied to.
- Rejection letters. There are many polite formulas of letting you know that your paper is not going to be published in a particular journal. These letters are instantly understood and since they do not need to be replied to, no time needs to be wasted on them from an idiomatic point of view.

We have divided up the letters to editors into:

- Submission letters
- Re-submission letters
- Re-configuration letters
- Letters of thanks for an invitation to publish an article in a journal
- Letters asking about the status of a paper
- Other letters

Submission Letters

Submission letters are quite easy to write since the main message to convey is the type and title of the paper you are submitting and the name of the corresponding author. Many standard letters can be used for this purpose and we do not think you have to waste too much time on them. For the most part, they are preliminary material that just needs to be sent along with the paper itself.

R. Ribes et al., *English for Biomedical Scientists,*
DOI: 10.1007/978-3-540-77127-2_5, © Springer-Verlag Berlin Heidelberg 2009

Editors of scientific journals need to deal with huge numbers of manuscripts. Thus, submission letters must be kept particularly brief. Nevertheless, in some instances you may want to add a paragraph to highlight the main message of your work or its particular suitability for the journal. Such brief comments may help getting the editor's attention.

Ricardo Palomino M.D, Ph.D.
The Anthony Nolan Research Institute
London, United Kingdom
rpalomino@rfc.ucl.ac.uk

April 11, 2002

Dr. Nicholas Silverman
European Editor
Journal of Gene Therapy

Dear Dr. Silverman,

Please consider the manuscript entitled *"Functional impairment of human T-lymphocytes following retroviral transduction: Implications for gene therapy"* for publication in the *Journal of Gene Therapy*.

The immune competence of retrovirus-mediated gene modified T-cells is critical for a beneficial effect to follow their adoptive transfer into patients. In this study, we show a functional disadvantage for PHA-expanded cells in their capacity to respond in vitro to allogeneic and viral-specific stimulation. Also, we identify alternative transduction protocols that preserve this functional capacity, and uncover the underlying mechanisms that may explain these functional differences. We believe that the *Journal of Gene Therapy*, which particularly encourages clinical applications of gene therapy techniques, would be a most suitable journal to communicate this work that we submit for your consideration.

Thank you very much for your time and consideration. We look forward to hearing from you soon.

Yours sincerely,

Ricardo Palomino

Re-submission Letters

Re-submission letters must thoroughly address the comments and suggestions of acceptance letters. In these letters, the corresponding author must let the editor know that all, or at least most, of the suggested changes have been made and, in so doing, the paper could be ready for publication. These letters do play an important role in the acceptance or rejection of a paper. Sometimes a lack of fluency in English prevents the corresponding author conveying the corrections made in the manuscript and the reasons why other suggested changes were not made.

Let's review the following example:

Dear Dr. Ho,

First of all, we would like to thank you for the opportunity to present an improved version of our paper for consideration for publication in the journal. After a thorough review of the reviewers' comments, we are now submitting a modified manuscript, "*Standardized MRI evaluation of hepatic iron overload*" for re-evaluation.

In response to the general comments, we have now included:
– New examples and electronic format to improve overall quality of the images presented.
– An imaging-based diagnostic algorithm for the diagnosis and follow-up of iron overload of the liver (new Tables 2 and 3).

In addition you can find a point-by-point rebuttal to all other points raised by the reviewers in the appendix attached to this letter.

We hope this new version will now be suitable for publication in the journal.

Yours sincerely,

Antonio Belafonte, MD, and co-authors

Re-configuration Letters

Sometimes the paper is accepted provided its configuration is changed, i.e., from a pictorial review to a pictorial essay. Re-configuration letters are re-submission letters as well and, therefore, tend to be long.

As we carry on looking at types of letters, we will also provide you with basic rules and recommendations. Review this example from which we have extracted and underlined several sentences for practical reference.

"Functional impairment of human T-lymphocytes following PHA-induced expansion and retroviral transduction: Implications for gene therapy" (JGT: 02-1343)

Dear Dr. Silverman, *(1)*

We have re-configured our manuscript referenced above*(2)* in the form of a Brief Report following your suggestion*(3)* and we have made as many changes as possible with regard to the reviewers' recommendations taking into account the space limitation imposed by the new format of the paper*(4)*.

We have tried to combine the data presented into a smaller number of figures, as required, and have given priority to the most relevant figures, the data of which cannot be described in the text*(5)*. The re-configuration of the manuscript has shortened it so drastically that we have had to rewrite it entirely and for this reason we do not attach an annotated copy*(6)* – if you still consider this necessary please let us know*(7)*. We have included in the new version a single table with statistical analysis data to "allow the reader to more easily reach the information shortening the length of the manuscript text"*(8)*as stated by reviewer no. 2*(9)* in his general remarks.

The major changes in our manuscript are:

1. *The title has been modified to* "Functional impairment of human T-lymphocytes following PHA-induced expansion and retroviral transduction: Implications for gene therapy" following your recommendation*(10)*.
2. We have included the technical parameters of our imaging protocol although it has not been possible to expand the technical section as suggested by reviewer no. 1*(11)* due to space limitation.
3. Similarly, the description of the methodology has been referenced to prior publications because the text could not be expanded as suggested by reviewer no. 2 due to space limitation*(12)*.
4. With regard to figures*(13)*:
   a. We have overall deleted two of the original figures.
   b. The raw dot-plot data have been incorporated*(14)*, as suggested, in figures 3 and 4.
   c. The image quality of figure 2 has been improved*(15)*.

5. We have assigned distinct figures to different entities in most cases although the limited number of figures allowed - 15 - made it impossible to do it in allc ases.
6. With regard to comments on figures 1 and 2 by reviewer no. 1*(16)*:
   - Figure 1a does indeed show the healthy controls data*(17)*. Aortic enhancement is not well seen due to the poor contrast resolution of this image which was acquired a long time ago and was one of our first abdominal MR 3D acquisitions.
   - Figure 2c shows confocal imaging as described in the revised version of the legend*(18)*
7. Results and Discussion sections in the manuscript have been combined as required by the new format*(19)*.

We look forward to hearing from you,*(20)*

Yourss incerely, *(21)*

Ricardo Palomino, MD, and co-authors*(22)*

1. *Dear Dr. Silverman,*
   - This sentence ends with a comma rather than a semicolon.
2. *We have reconfigured the manuscript referenced above*
   - The content of the letter must be summarized in the first paragraph.
3. *... following your suggestion*
   - This is one of the commonest sentences in re-submission/re-configuration letters.
4. *... space limitation imposed by the new format of the paper*
   - Space limitation, provided the new format limits it, must be taken into consideration by both the authors and the reviewers.
5. *have given priority to the most relevant figures, the data of which cannot be described in the text*
   - May be a criterion for the shortening of the manuscript.
6. *for this reason we do not attach an annotated copy*
   - Whenever you don't follow a suggestion, you must give an explanation.
7. *if you still consider it necessary please let us know*
   - Always leave open the possibility of adding more information in further correspondence.
8. *"allow the reader to more easily reach the information shortening the length of the manuscript text"*
   - You can use as an argument what was literally suggested by the reviewer by writing it in inverted commas.
9. *as stated by reviewer no. 2*
   - This is a usual way of addressing a reviewer's comment.
10. *... following your recommendation*
    - This is also a usual way of addressing a reviewer's comment.

11. *We have included the technical parameters of our imaging protocol as suggested by reviewer no. 1*
    – This is a usual way of addressing a reviewer's comment.
12. *Similarly, … could not be expanded as suggested by reviewer no. 2 due to space limitation*
    – Whenever you don't follow a suggestion, you must give an explanation.
13. *With regard to figures:*
    – Or regarding figures, as regards figures, as for figures (without the preposition "to").
14. *The raw dot-plot data have been incorporated*
    – This is a usual way of addressing a reviewer's comment.
15. *The image quality of figure 2 has been improved*
    – This is a usual way of addressing a reviewer's comment.
16. *With regard to comments on figures 1 and 2 by reviewer no. 1:*
    – This is a usual way of addressing a reviewer's comment.
17. *Figure 1a does indeed show the healthy controls data*
    – This is a usual way of addressing a reviewer's comment.
18. *Figure 2c shows confocal imaging as described in the revised version of the legend*
    – This is a usual way of addressing a reviewer's comment.
19. *Results and Discussion sections in the manuscript have been combined as required by the new format*
    – This is a usual way of addressing a reviewer's comment.
20. *We look forward to hearing from you*
    – Remember that the verb following the verb "to look forward to" must be in its -*ing* form.
21. *Yourss incerely,*
    – Bear in mind that if you don't know the name of the editor you should write "Yours faithfully" instead.
22. *Ricardo Palomino, MD, and co-authors*
    – Although the corresponding author is the only one who signs the letter, sometimes a reference is made to the co-authors.

Letters of Thanks for an Invitation to Publish an Article in a Journal

These are simple and usually short letters in which we let the editor of a journal know how pleased we are regarding his/her invitation and how much we appreciate his/her consideration.

Your address   Date

Receiver's name and address

Dear Dr. Massa,

Thank you for the invitation to submit a manuscript on T-cell function following retroviral transduction. We have recently presented in the meeting of the European Association for Gene Therapy data from our lab on new molecular mechanisms of the effects of retroviral transduction on lymphocyte proliferation and functional maturation.

Please find the abstract with that data attached.

If you think this would be of interest for the monographic number that you described we'd be happy to participate in the project. Please advise us in terms of number of words and figures and overall style of the manuscript for publication.

I look forward to hearing from you.

Yours sincerely,

A. J. Cantona, MD

Asking About the Status of a Paper

In these letters we inquire about the situation of our article since we have not received any response from the journal. Regrettably in the academic world "no news" is not usually "good news", and many of these inquiries end up with a polite rejection letter.

Dear Dr. Ross,

As I have not received any response regarding the manuscript "Sox10 determines oligodendrocyte development in the mouse," I wondered whether you could give us any feed-back on the status of the paper.

Please use the following e-mail address for further correspondence:

sanzzap@seram.es

I look forward to hearing from you at your earliest convenience.

Yourss incerely,

J. Sanz, MD, PhD

Other Letters

Asking for Permission to Use Someone's Name as a Referee

Platero Heredia, 19
Córdoba 14012
SPAIN

17 April 2006

John G. Adams, MD
Department of Cell Biology
Harvard Medical School
22 Beacon St
Boston, MA, USA

Dear Dr. Adams,

I am applying for a post as Assistant Professor at the Department of Biology at Universidad Autónoma, Madrid (Spain). International references from world leaders in my field would be of great help. You may remember that we had the opportunity to interact on multiple occasions and work together in a number of projects during my time in Dr. Styles lab in Boston. I should be most grateful if, from this frame of reference, you allowed me to use your name as a referee.

Yourss incerely,

Guido Andreotti, MD

Postponing the Commencement of Duties

Gran Vía, 113
Madrid, 28004
Spain

17 November 2006

Robert H. Shaw, MD
Department of Genetics
Massachusetts General Hospital
22 Beacon St
Boston, MA, USA

Dear Dr. Shaw,

I would like to thank you for your letter of 11 February 2001 offering me an Instructor position in your lab from April 1st, 2001.

I am very pleased to accept the post but unfortunately I will not be able to arrive to Boston until middle of April due to an expected delay in the processing of my J1 visa. Would it, therefore, be possible for you to postpone the commencement of my duties to the second fortnight of April?

I look forward to hearing from you.

Yourss incerely,

Angela Maldini, MD

In Summary

To sum up, a few simple formal details must be recalled:

- "Dear Dr. Smith," is the usual way to begin an academic letter. Recall that after the name of the editor you must insert a comma or nothing at all. Continue the letter with a new paragraph.
- The usual formula "find enclosed ..." can nowadays be replaced by "find attached ..." taking into consideration that most papers are submitted via the internet.
- "I look forward to hearing from you" is a standard sentence at the end of any formal letter and you have to bear in mind, in order to avoid a usual mistake, that "to" is a preposition to be followed by a gerund rather than the infinitive particle of the verb that follows it. Do not make the usual mistake of writing "I look forward to hear from you." Similar formulas are: "I look forward to receiving your comments on ..."
- "Your consideration is appreciated" or "Thank you for your consideration" are standard sentences to be written at the end of letters to editors.
- "I look forward to receiving your feedback on ..." is a slightly more casual formula commonly used in letters to editors.
- "Yours faithfully," is used when you do not know the name of the person you are writing to, whereas "Sincerely,"/"Sincerely yours,"/"Yours sincerely," must be written when you address the letter to a person by name. Therefore, if the letter begins with "Dear Dr. Olsen," it must end up with "Yours sincerely," and if it is addressed to the editor as such it must finish with "Yours faithfully,". Other appropriate common expressions are "With best wishes," or "With kind regards,". Don't forget to add your signature below the adverb or pronoun.
- Remember that dates are written differently in American (month-day-year) and British English (day-month-year).
- Whenever you cannot address one of the editors' suggestions, explain why it was not possible in the re-submission letter so the reviewers do not waste time looking for it in the manuscript. For example:
  - *We have included the technical parameters of our imaging protocol although it has not been possible to expand the technical section as suggested by reviewer no. 1 due to space limitation.*

UNIT VI

Unit VI   Attending a Scientific Course or Conference

Introduction

In the following pages we take a look inside international scientific meetings. We recommend upper-intermediate English speakers to quickly go over them and intermediate English speakers to review this section thoroughly in order to become familiar with the jargon of international congresses, as well as that of the conversational scenarios such as the airport, plane, customs, taxi, hotel checking in, and finally the course itself that make up the usual itinerary of every scientist attending an international course.

Most beginners do not go alone to their first courses abroad. This fact would appear to be a relief for non-natives, who do not need to cope with the idiomatic difficulties on their own. In reality, it has an important drawback: most non native English-speaking scientists in training go back to their countries of origin having uttered hardly a single word in English. There is no doubt that speaking in English with your fellow countrymen in an international meeting is unnatural. That much we'll give you. But the sad reality is that you are very likely to spend over 90% of your time talking with the very colleagues that you came to the meeting with and about the same things you were talking about back home. So, what is the point of traveling then? Scary thought, isn't it? Our heartfelt advice, if you feel brave and radical enough to go for it, is that you kindly lose them! That's correct. Go interact with the rest of the crowd. It'll surely be tougher at first, but infinitely more rewarding. Do not waste such an excellent opportunity to improve and maintain your level of both colloquial English and scientific English.

The pressure to get your English up to scratch (i.e., up to the standard required or expected) is even greater if you happen to be making a presentation at the meeting. Most non-native English-speaking lecturers resign themselves to just giving the lecture and ... "survive," forgetting that if they do not enjoy their lecture, the audience will not enjoy it either. They think that to enjoy giving a lecture, your native tongue must be English. We strongly disagree with this point since many speakers do not enjoy their talks in their own native tongues, and it is our understanding that having a good time delivering a presentation has much more to do with your approach to it and your personality than with your native tongue.

R. Ribes et al., *English for Biomedical Scientists*,
DOI: 10.1007/978-3-540-77127-2_6, © Springer-Verlag Berlin Heidelberg 2009

Interacting with international colleagues is certainly a good way to warm up to a good presentation in English as a second language. Don't let your lack of fluency in day-to-day English in any way undermine your ability to deliver a good or even great presentation. Unit 7 will discuss in detail how to improve your presentation, feel at ease giving it, and even enjoy it. This unit now provides you with tips and useful sentences in your itinerary to an international scientific course: airport, plane, customs, taxi, hotel checking in, and finally, the course itself. Unless you have overcome the conversational hurdles in the scenarios that come before the course, firstly, you are not going to get to the course venue and, secondly, if you do get to it, you will not feel like delivering your presentation.

Travel and Hotel Arrangements

Airport

Getting to the Airport

- How can I get to the airport?
- How soon should we be at the airport before take-off?

Checking in

- May I have your passport and flight tickets, please? Of course, here you are.
- Are you Mr. Vida? Right, I am. How do you spell it? V-I-D-A (rehearse the spelling of your last name since if it is not an English one, you are going to be asked about its spelling many times).
- Here is your boarding card. Your flight leaves from gate 43. Thank you.
- You are only allowed two carry-on items. You'll have to check in that larger bag.

Questions a Passenger Might Ask

- I want to fly to London leaving this afternoon. Is there a direct flight? Is it via Zurich?
- Is it direct? Yes, it is direct/No, it is one-stop.
- Is there a stop-over? Yes, you have a stop-over in Berlin.
- How long is the stop-over? About 1 hour.
- Do I have to change planes? Yes, you have to change planes at …
- How much carry-on luggage am I allowed?
- What weight am I allowed?
- My luggage is overweight. How much more do I need to pay?
- Is a meal served? Yes, lunch will be served during the flight.

- What time does the plane to Chicago leave?
- When does the next flight to Chicago leave?
- Can I get onto the next flight?
- Can I change my flight schedule?
- What's the departure time?
- Is the plane on time?
- What's the arrival time?
- Will I be able to make my connection?
- I have misplaced my hand luggage. Where is lost property?
- How much is it to upgrade this ticket to first class?
- I want to change the return flight date from Boston to Madrid to November 30th.
- Is it possible to purchase an open ticket?
- I have missed my flight to New York. When does the next flight leave, please?
- Can I use the ticket I have or do I need to pay for a new one?

Announcing Changes in an Airline Flight

- Our flight to Madrid has been cancelled because of snow.
- Our flight to Chicago has been delayed; however, all connecting flights can be made.
- Flight number 112 to Paris has been cancelled.
- Flight number 1145 has been moved to gate B12.
- Passengers for flight number 112 to London go to gate 7. Hurry up! Our flight has been called over the loudspeaker.

At the Boarding Gate

- We will begin boarding soon.
- We are now boarding passengers in rows 24 through 36.
- May I see your boarding card?

Arrival

- Pick up your luggage at the terminal.
- Where can I find a luggage cart (*UK*, trolley)?
- Where is the taxi stand (*UK*, taxi rank)?
- Where is the subway stop (*UK*, underground station)?
- Where is the way out?

Complaining About Lost or Damaged Luggage

- My luggage is missing.
- One of my bags seems to be missing.
- My luggage is damaged.
- One of my suitcases has been lost.

Exchange Office

- Where is the exchange office?
- What is the rate for the American Dollar?
- Could you change 1000 Euros into American Dollars?

Customs and Immigration Control

- May I see your passport, please?
- Do you have your visa?
- What is your nationality?
- What is the purpose of your journey? The purpose of my journey is a holiday, touring, family affairs, studying …
- How long do you plan on staying?
- Empty your pockets and put your wallet, keys, cellular phone (*UK*, mobile phone), and coins on this tray.
- Remove any metallic objects you are carrying and put them on this tray.
- Openy our laptop.
- Take off your shoes. Put them in this tray too.
- Do you have anything to declare? No, I don't have anything to declare.
- Do you have anything to declare? No, I only have personal effects.
- Do you have anything to declare? Yes, I am a doctor and I'm carrying some surgical instruments.
- Do you have anything to declare? Yes, I have bought six bottles of whisky and four cartons of cigarettes in the duty free shop.
- How much currency are you bringing into the country? I haven't got any foreignc urrency.
- Open your bag, please.
- I need to examine the contents of your bag.
- May I close my bag? Sure.
- Please place your suitcases on the table.
- What do you have in these parcels? Some presents for my wife and kids.
- How much duty do I have to pay?
- Where is the exchange office?

During the Flight

Very few exchanges are likely during a normal flight. If you are familiar with them you will realize how fluency interferes positively with your mood. Conversely, if you need a pillow and are not able to ask for one, your self-confidence will shrink, your neck will hurt, and you will not ask for anything else during the flight. On my first flight to the States I did not know how to ask for a pillow and tried to convince myself that I did not actually need one. When I looked it up in my guide, asked for it, and the stewardess brought the pillow, I gladly and pleasantly fell asleep.

Do not let lack of fluency spoil an otherwise perfect flight.

- Is there an aisle/window seat free? (I asked for one at the check-in and they told me I should ask on board just in case there had been a cancellation.)
- Excuse me, you are in my seat. Oh! Sorry, I didn't notice.
- Fasten your seat belt, please.
- Your life-jacket is under your seat.
- Smoking is not allowed during the flight.
- Please would you bring me a blanket/pillow?
- Is there a business class seat free?
- Can I upgrade to first class on board?
- Would you like a cup of coffee/tea/a glass of soda? A glass of soda, please.
- What would you prefer, chicken or beef/fish or meat? Beef/Fish, please.
- Is there a vegetarian menu?
- Stewardess, I'm not feeling well. Do you have anything for flight sickness? Could you bring me another sick bag, please?
- Stewardess, I have a headache. Do you have an aspirin?
- Stewardess, this gentleman is disturbing me.

In the Taxi (*US* Cab)

Think for a moment about taking a taxi in your city. How many sentences do you suppose would be exchanged in normal, and even extraordinary, conditions? I assure you that with fewer than two dozen sentences you will solve more than ninety per cent of possible situations.

Asking Where to Get a Taxi

- Where is the nearest taxi stand (*UK*, taxi rank)?
- Where can I get a taxi/taxicab/cab?

Basic Instructions

- Hi, take me downtown/to the Sheraton hotel, please.
- Please would you take me to the Airport?
- It is rush hour; I don't go to the airport.
- Sorry, I am not on duty.
- It will cost you double fare to leave the city.
- I need to go to the Convention Center.
- Which way do you want me to take you, via Fifth or Seventh Avenue? Either one would be OK.
- Is there any surcharge to the airport?

Concerning Speed in a Taxi

- To downtown as quick as you can.
- Are you in a hurry? Yes, I'm in a hurry.
- I'm late; please hurry.
- Slowd own!
- Do you have to drive so fast? There is no need to hurry. I am not in a rush at all.

Concerning Smoking in a Taxi

- Would you mind putting your cigarette out?
- Would you mind not smoking, please?

Asking to Stop and Wait

- Stop at number 112, please.
- Which side of the street?
- Do you want me to drop you at the door?
- Pull over; I'll be back in a minute.
- Please wait here a minute.
- Stop here.

Concerning the Temperature in a Taxi

- Would you please wind your window up? It's a bit cold.
- Could you turn the heat up/down/on/off?
- Could you turn the air conditioning on/off?
- Is the air conditioning/heating on?

Payment

- How much is it?
- How much do I owe you?
- Is the tip included?
- Do you have change for a twenty/fifty (dollar bill)? Sorry, I don't (have any change).
- Keep the change.
- Would you give me a receipt?
- I need a receipt, please.
- I think that is too expensive.
- They have never charged me this before. Give me a receipt, please. I think I'll make a complaint.
- Can I pay by credit card? Sure, swipe your card here.

At the Hotel

Checking In

- May I help you?
- Hello, I have reserved a room under the name of Dr. Viamonte.
- For how many people? Two, my wife and I.
- Do you need my ID?
- Do you need my credit card?
- How long will you be staying? We are staying for a week.
- You will have to wait until your room is ready.
- Here is your key.
- Enjoy your stay. Thank you.
- Is there anybody who can help me with my bags?
- Do you need a bellboy? Yes, please.
- I'll have someone bring your luggage up.

Preferences

- Can you double-check that we have a double room with a view of the beach/city …?
- I would like a room at the front/at the rear.
- I would like the quietest room you have.
- I would like a non-smoking room.
- I would like a suite.
- How many beds? I want a double bed/a single bed.
- I asked for two single beds.
- I'd like a king-sized bed.
- I'd like a queen-sized bed.
- We will need a crib (*UK*, cot) for the baby.
- Are all of your rooms en suite? Yes, all of our rooms have a bath or shower.
- Is breakfast included?
- Does the hotel have a car park?
- Do you have a parking lot (*UK*, car park) nearby?

The Stay

- Can you give me a wake-up call at seven every morning?
- There is no hot water. Would you please send someone to fix it?
- The TV is not working properly. Would you please send someone to fix it?
- The bathtub has no plug. Would you please send someone up with one.
- The people in the room next to mine are making a racket. Would you please tell them to keep it down?
- I want to change my room. It's too noisy.

- What time does breakfast start?
- How can I get to the city center?
- Can we change Euros into Canadian Dollars?
- Could you recommend a good restaurant near to the hotel?
- Could you recommend a good restaurant?
- Would you give me the number for room service?
- I will have a cheese omelet, a ham sandwich, and an orange juice.
- Are there vending machines available?
- Do you have a fax machine available?
- Do you serve meals?
- Is there a pool/restaurant ...?
- How do I get room service?
- Is there wireless/internet connection?
- The sink is clogged.
- The toilet is running.
- The toilet is leaking.
- My toilet overflowed!
- The toilet doesn't flush.
- The bath is leaking.
- My bathroom is flooded.
- The bath faucets (*UK*, taps) drip day and night.
- The water is rust-colored.
- The pipes are always banging.
- The water is too hot.
- The water is never hot enough.
- I don't have any hot water.

Checking Out

- How much is it?
- Do you accept credit cards?
- Can I pay in Dollars/Euros?
- I'd like a receipt, please.
- What time is checkout? Checkout is at 11 a.m.
- I would like to check out.
- Is there a penalty for late checkout?
- Please would you have my luggage brought down?
- Would you please call me a taxi?
- How far is the nearest bus stop/subway station?

Complaints

- Excuse me, there is a mistake on the receipt:
- I have had only one breakfast.
- I thought breakfast was included.

- I have been in a single room.
- Have you got a complaints book?
- Please would you give me my car keys?
- Is there anybody here who can help me with my luggage?

Course Example

General Information

By way of example let's review some general information concerning a course program, focusing on those terms that may not be known by beginners.

Language

The official language of the course will be English.

Dress Code

Formal dress is required for the Opening Ceremony and for the Social Dinner. Casual wear is acceptable for all other events and occasions (although formal dress is customary for lecturers).

Commercial Exhibition

Participants will have the opportunity to visit representatives from pharmaceutical, diagnostic and biotech companies, and publishers at their stands to discuss new developments and receive up-to-date product information.

Although most beginners don't talk to salespeople due to their lack of fluency in English, talking to salespeople in commercial stands is a good way to practice scientific English and, by the same token, receive up-to-date information on equipment and devices you currently use, or will use in the future, at your institution.

Disclosure Statements

You need to be aware that in recent years, an increasing focus is being put on the need for medical and biomedical scientists not only to avoid, but to actively disclose any significant relationships with industry that may result in a conflict of interest. Many professional societies are putting enforcement mechanisms in place to ensure that oral and poster presentations at their annual congresses fully disclose conflicts of interest.

A conflict of interest may exist when professionals have material interests, regardless of their value, that could influence or be perceived by others as influencing their professional actions and decisions. Conflicts of interest are relevant not only to relationship between physicians and pharmaceutical industry, but also to other phases of biomedical research, including pre-clinical research.

We list below a number of activities involving the industry and the volunteer (from volunteer self-disclosure), partner or spouse, which are susceptible to conflict of interest disclosure:

- Employment
- Scientific advisory board membership
- Board of directors membership
- Consultancy
- Participating in company-sponsored speakers' bureaus
- Expert testimony
- Any other form of honoraria
- Research funding
- Accepting subsidies for the cost of traveling to meetings.

Faculty

Name and current posts of the speakers:

- Russel J. Curtin, MD. Cell Biology. Division of Neurodevelopmental Biology, Beath Israel Deaconess Medical Center, Boston, MA

Guest Faculty

Name and current posts of speakers coming from institutions other than those organizing the course:

- Fergus B Schwartz, Professor of Medicine, New York School of Medicine; New York University Medical Center, New York, NY

How to Reach …

Arrival by plane

The international airport is situated about 25 kilometers outside the city. To reach the city center you can use the:

- City airport train. Every half-hour. Non-stop. 18 minutes from the airport direct to downtown, and from downtown direct to the airport. Fare: single, EUR 10; return, EUR 18.
- Regional railway, line 6. Travel time: 36 minutes. Frequency: every 30 minutes. Fare: single, EUR 12; return, EUR 20. Get off at "Charles Square". From there use the underground line "U7" to "Park Street".
- Bus. International Airport to … Charles Square. Travel time: 25 minutes. Fare: EUR 8.
- Taxi. There is a taxi stand to the south of the arrival hall. A taxi to the city center costs around EUR 45 (depending on traffic).

Arrival by Train
For detailed information about the timetable you can call …

At the railway station you can use the underground to reach the city.

Congress venue (where the course is to be held, e.g., hotel, university, convention center …):

Continental Hotel
32 Park Street, 23089 …
Phone: … /Fax: …
E-mail: continentalhotel@hhs.com

To reach the venue from the city centre (Charles Square) take the U1 underground line (green). Leave the train at Park Street and take the exit marked Continental Hotel. Traveling time: approximately 10 minutes.

Weather

The weather in … in December is usually cold with occasional snow. The daytime temperatures normally range from $-5°$ to $+5°C$.

Registration

Generally you will have been registered beforehand and you will not have to register at the course's registration counter. If you do have to register at the congress venue, the following are some of the most usual exchanges that may take place during registration:

Attendee:	May I have a registration form, please?
Course attendant:	Do you want me to fill it out (*UK*, fill it in) for you? Are you an ECR member? Are you attending the full course?
Trainee:	No. I'm a graduate student and I have applied for a trainee scholarship.
Course attendant:	Can I have your ID and see your chairman's confirmation letter?
Trainee:	I was told it was faxed last week. Would you check that, please?
Attendee:	I'll pay by cash/credit card. Charge it to my credit card. Would you make out an invoice?
Course attendant:	Do you need an invoice? Do you want me to draw up an invoice?
Attendee:	Where should I get my badge?
Course attendant:	Join that line (*UK*, queue).

Registration fees and deadlines

	Until 13 November 2006	After 13 November 2006
Full fee member	€ 330.-	€ 450.-
Full fee non-member	€ 540.-	€ 650.-
Graduate student	€ 190.-	€ 260.-
Technician/Research Assistant*	€ 140.-	€ 180.-
University administrator*	€ 140.-	€ 180.-
Single-day ticket	On-site only	€ 240.-
Single half-day ticket(Tuesday only)	On-site only	€ 80.-
Weekend ticket(Saturday 07:00 to Sunday 18:00)	On-site only	€ 360.-
Industry day ticket	On-site only	€ 90.-

Course Planning

The basic idea whenever you attend an international scientific course is that you must rehearse beforehand those situations that are inevitably going to happen and, in so doing, you will keep to a minimum embarrassing situations catching you off-guard. Just a few words, set phrases, and collocations must be known in this environment and we can assure you that knowing them will give you the confidence needed to make your participation in the course a personal success.

The first piece of advice is: read the program of the course thoroughly and look up in the dictionary or ask your more experienced colleagues about the words and concepts you don't know. Since the program is available before the course starts, go over it at home; you don't need to read the scientific program at the course's venue.

"Adjourn" is one of those typical program terms with which one gets familiar once the session is "adjourned." Although many could think that most terms are going to be integrated and understood by their context, our intention is to go over those "insignificant" terms that may prevent you from optimizing your time at the course.

An example of a course plan is presented in Table 1. The course plan may contain the following elements:

- *Satellite symposia*: Scientific events sponsored by pharmaceutical or biotechnology firms where new drugs (mainly contrast media), techniques or devices are presented to the scientific community.
- *Plenary sessions*: These events usually take place at midday gathering all participants around outstanding members of the scientific community.
- *Educational sessions*: Important scientific topics are presented with an educational purpose covering various aspects of the field.

- *Special focus sessions*: The aim of a special focus session is to deal with a relevant "hot topic," presented in such a way as to promote debate between the panelists and the audience.
- *Oral scientific sessions*: The Scientific Committee selects, from all the abstracts submitted, the most outstanding research work and invites the authors to make a presentation of their methods and conclusions (usually not longer than 10–15 minutes). A round of questions and/or comments is usually permitted.
- *Poster sessions*: Quality abstracts that do not make it to the oral sessions will be presented as posters. The presenting author will need to stand by the poster to discuss it with any members of the audience interested. Although oral presentations tend to select somewhat higher score quality abstracts, a poster might be far more useful in terms of time to interact with colleagues and opportunities for (and ease of) exchange of experiences and opinions. Rehearse for your poster too. If your data is good, you will certainly have people coming along with questions. Being ready will give you the chance to make the most out of your presentation.
- *Adjourn*: Close (break or recess) at the end of a session.

Unit VII   Giving Presentations for Biomedical Scientists

As a biomedical scientist you will have to present your quality research at international conferences, the vast majority of which are run in English. International scientific conferences are in a universe all of their own. In this universe, attendees and speakers come from many different countries with their own cultures and consequently their own habits in terms of behavior and public speaking. However, most speakers set aside, at least partially, their cultural identity to embrace the international medical conference style. This standardization is part of the globalization that we are all witnessing.

As part of the globalization of biomedical science, many international non-native scientists will go to English-speaking countries to complete training and work. In this case, and even before they make it to presenting in international meetings, they will have to face lab meetings, departmental retreats, university PhD student sessions, all of which will logically be run in English.

The most widely spoken language in international conferences and by international scientists in general is not Chinese, Spanish, Japanese, or French anymore. It is not even standard English, but the new phenomenon of broken English. This language is the result of simplifying English to make it as neutral and understandable as possible, removing colloquial idioms, regional expressions, or any other source of linguistic confusion.

In this new universe, you will find yourself having to make a conscious effort to adapt to these explicit and implicit rules. Some of them are discussed in the following sections.

Having read this chapter you will not only be able to improve your presentations or feel at ease giving them, but you might also actually end up being able to convey your message and, who knows? … you might even enjoy it. There is no reason why the language barrier cannot be overcome to give you the opportunity to be as good a communicator in English as you are in your own language.

Know Your Audience

The whole point of giving a scientific talk, or any talk for that matter, is to convey a message to an audience. You must therefore put your audience first. Learning about them is the first step and the best way to get the layout of your message

R. Ribes et al., *English for Biomedical Scientists*,
DOI: 10.1007/978-3-540-77127-2_7, © Springer-Verlag Berlin Heidelberg 2009

right. This principle applies to any speaker, but it can be a source of particular confidence and sense of safety for non-native scientists having to present their data in English. What is it that you should know about the audience then? As a minimum, you should find out:

- Who they are and what brings them to your presentation:
  - Are they BSc students approaching their first hands-on experience in a lab and counting on you for a warm-up introduction?
  - Are they fellow lab mates wanting to learn some more specific technical and experimental details from your last set of experiments?
  - Are they potential employers or colleagues in a lab that you are applying to trying to figure out how good a candidate you are?
  - Are they general attendees at an international conference that you are presenting your results at?
  - Are they a grant committee that is going to decide on the continuation of your research support grant?
- How many of them will be there:
  - A small group that facilitates a closer level of complicity about the message?
  - A huge auditorium with a barely recognizable sea of faces that may call for a somewhat more formal style?
- How familiar they are with your topic:
  - How much of a general background introduction would they need to follow the rest?
- → Think about who your audience is, what they are expecting from you, how much they know about the topic of your presentation and you'll be ready to put together a main message to convey to them.

Choose a Relevant Main Message

Once you know your audience, you must use that knowledge to choose a central message for your presentation that is relevant to them. We all understand the difficulty to fit all your data, all your results, all that you know and could tell about your topic of research into a mere 15, 30 or even 45 minutes. Well, squeezing in everything you can tell about your topic should actually never be your goal. Beware of the extent of your knowledge. It might work against the clarity and the interest of your presentation.

In addition to scientific information, some lecturers tend to give too much minor detail in their presentations. Their introduction is often full of information that is of little relevance to the international audience (for example, the name, date, and code of local, provincial, regional, and national laws regulating laboratory standards in his/her institution; or even the background information on the main researchers of a trial including their graduation year and shoe size … or a full history of the 16th century building where the research centre stands today and subsequent restorations it has undergone, etc). In these cases, by the time all these details have been given and the presentation has passed the introduction stage, time is up and the chairperson starts making desperate signs to the speaker. Even worse, the audience may be lost and have no idea of what the talk is actually about.

Our practical advice is that once you have chosen a central message which is relevant to your audience, you should list and select a small number of critical points to convey it, and maybe list some additional points to reinforce it if time permits. Be critical with yourself. Examine your reasons to include every particular point. Remember that it is your audience that you should have in mind when producing your presentation.

- Is it you who finds a particular point or argument interesting, or your audience that needs to know it?
- Is the point indispensable to support your central message or only useful to reinforce it?
- Does the point bring the audience's attention towards the central message or into a secondary, less relevant discussion?

Put Together Your Presentation: Structure and Delivery

Once you know your audience and what you are going to tell them, you are ready to plan the delivery of the message. For an effective delivery, the points in your talk will have to be built into a structure that guides the audience through and keeps their attention. If your presentation has no structure, the audience won't follow you. The type of structure depends on the type of data, on the audience and the setting as discussed above, and ultimately, on the speaker. The structure of your presentation is your choice. As long as it is logical and adapts to your needs (i.e., your audience's) any type of structure will probably do the job. One of the more widely accepted and simple structures proposed to make a presentation good reads as follows:

1. Say what you are going to say
2. Say it
3. Say what you just said

We will use this model to help you put together your presentation and provide you with practical advice and examples.

1. Say what you are going to say (i.e., Introduction)

Just imagine that you have to deliver your presentation in the *graveyard slot* (the graveyard slot is the first presentation after the lunch-break, when most of the audience will be suffering from postprandial somnolence and very likely you will not hear a sound except for that of snores). Of course, you would want to greet the audience and to thank whoever invited you to talk. But even so, job number one is to awaken the audience's attention, to give them an idea of what you're going to tell them and why it is relevant for them – *say what you are going to say.*

This applies to all presentations. You must make the start of your presentation stand out from a monotonous string of talks in a conference as much as from postprandial somnolence in order to engage your audience. At a minimum, your introduction must include:

- The main message of your talk
- An estimation of the time the talk is going to take
  → *In the next 30 minutes I would like to show you recent data from our lab showing that regulatory T-cells play an important role in anti-tumor responses following allogeneic transplantation, and may be used as a useful novel tool to predict the risk of disease relapse in these patients.*

- A very general overview of how the data will be presented
  → *I am going to start by briefly summarizing the current understanding of the role of regulatory T-cells in allogeneic transplantation, from where our study takes off. Then, I will show you our recent data on the role of these cells on anti-tumor responses in vivo in a murine model of transplantation for leukemia. Finally, I will conclude this presentation with recent findings in this area in humans, in a cohort of transplant recipients for hematological malignancies.*

Time is a very cultural thing. When addressing your audience at the beginning of a talk in English use:

- *Good morning:* from the start time to 12:00.
- *Good afternoon: from 12:01 onwards, even though your metabolism may be far from feeling afternoon-ish until your usual lunch time has gone by and is begging you to say "good morning."*
- Good evening: from 18:00 onwards. Note that if we have to give a presentation, make a speech, or offer a toast at 22:00, we should never begin with "good night;" that should be reserved only for when we are going to bed. So "good night" is not supposed to be said in public.

Useful Sentences for the Introduction of your Presentation
- Good morning. It is an honor to have the opportunity to speak to you about …
- Good afternoon. Thank you for your kind introduction. It is my pleasure to speak to you about an area of great interest to me.
- In the next few minutes I'll talk about …
- The topic I'll cover this afternoon is …

- In the next 20 minutes I'll show you ...
- In my talk on oligodendrocyte development, I want to share with you all our experience on ...
- Thank you for sticking around (informal way of addressing the last talk attendees).
- I'd like to thank Dr. Ho for his kind invitation.
- Thank you Dr. Wilson for inviting me to attend this course.
- Thank you Dr. Olsen. It is a great honor to be here talking about ...
- On behalf of my colleagues and assistants, I want to thank Dr. Smith for his kind invitation.
- I'd like to welcome you to this course on ... (to be said in the first talk of the course if you are a member of the organizing committee)
- Today, I want to talk to you about ...
- Now, allow me to introduce ...
- What I want to talk about this morning is ...
- During the next few minutes, I'd like to draw your attention to ...
- First of all, let me summarize the contents of my lecture on ...

2. Say it (i.e., Main Body of your presentation)

- But don't say it too fast or too slowly. In view of time constraints, there are various alternatives ranging from speaking as fast as the tongue can rattle, to cutting it down to 5 minutes and spending the other 15 minutes vacantly gazing at the audience. Every speaker develops a personal style over time, and the rhythm and speed of presentation is part of that style. American, British, and Australian scientists are often extremely fluent speakers (we know, we know ... they are using their mother tongue). However, remember that showing and commenting on five slides a minute and speaking faster than can be registered on a digital recorder will certainly never be a good way of conveying a message.
- Keep your language simple. Use short, concrete words and sentences rather than long, cumbersome ones. Use active rather than passive forms of the verbs. As a non-native-English speaker you will be making it easier on yourself. In addition, being concise is a common piece of advice also for native speakers.
- Break down the body of your presentation into several sections of data that can be connected. Every time you create a new ending and link it to a new beginning in the following section, the level of attention of the audience increases. If you set a dynamic pattern of beginnings and endings you will keep your audience connected to the data all the way through to the end of the presentation.

- Use the power of 3. The human mind is more prone to remember statements and facts that come in a list of three and build up to a climax. For example:
  - → *"Duty, honor, country. Those three hallowed words reverently dictate what you ought to be, what you can be, what you will be."* *(D. MacArthur)*
  - → *"Veni, vidi, vici."* *(Julius Cesar)*
  - → Say what you are going to say, say it, and then say what you just said (see above)

- Creativity and humor are always appreciated in a lecture hall … providing they are both appropriate and understood! So, make sure that your jokes can be understood internationally. We all know that humor is a very cultural thing, like time keeping, food preferences, etc. Some American speakers will start their presentation with a joke that most Europeans will not understand, not even the Irish or British. A British speaker will probably throw in the most sarcastic comment when you are least expecting it and in the same tone as if he or she were telling you about the mortality rate in his or her unit. A foreign (neither American nor British) scientist might just try to tell a long joke in English based on a play on words in his or her mother tongue which obviously doesn't work in English, and possibly involves religion, sport, and/or sex (as a general rule avoid religious and sex jokes in public presentations).

- Use visual aids to help you convey the message. The need for visual aid and the type depend on the type of talk. For the majority of proper scientific presentations, the audience expects certain information to be presented in certain ways. In addition, your organization or the venue where the presentation takes place may limit your choice in terms of type of equipment available or style and design of slides. In any case, there are a number of considerations you should always take into account:
  - Use visuals as your server, not your master. Don't let them get in between yourself and your audience. It's you and your message that you want the audience to take in and remember, not only your slides.
  - Don't ever say "sorry for this slide." Since you are the one who chooses the slides to be presented, get rid of those you would have to apologize for.
  - Don't hide behind long lists of graphics, diagrams, and tables. You should rather use part of your visuals to set the pace and rhythm of the presentation, to highlight the links between beginnings and endings of sections of data, to stimulate or even provoke your audience.
  - Don't read slides, but instead try to explain a few basic ideas as clearly as possible. Many intermediate English-speaking doctors and scientists find it hard to agree with this point because they can only feel some confidence if they read the presentation. Reading is the least-natural means of communicating experiences; we encourage you to present your paper without reading it. Although it will need much more intensive preparation, the delivery will be more fluid and – why not? – even brilliant. Many foreign doctors and scientists resign themselves to delivering just accept-

able talks and explicitly reject the possibility of making a presentation at the same level as they would in their own language. Do not reject the possibility of being as brilliant as you would be in your own language; the only difference is in the amount of rehearsal. Thorough rehearsal can provide you with amazing results; do not give up beforehand.

- Ask your audience questions; obviously not to check their knowledge, but rather as an instrument to increase their interest in a particular idea or link between sections of your presentation. Make sure that the questions are straightforward, simple, and with a clear answer or choice of an answer. As an alternative, rhetorical questions are easier and safer. They challenge and awaken the audience less, but won't leave you waiting for an answer in a silent room until you resume.
- Please do not read your presentation from a script. Even worse than reading from slides is to read from a script. An attempt to coordinate scribbled pages on the lectern with the slides in a presentation is a disaster waiting to happen. The worst consequence is that the audience will be paying attention to the noise of the passing pages and to the face of the speaker on the verge of a mental breakdown rather than to the presentation itself.
- Enjoy the show! When giving the presentation, relax; nobody knows more than you do about the specific subject that you are presenting. The only way to make people enjoy your presentation is by enjoying it yourself. You only have to communicate; being a good researcher or a competent scientist is not the same thing as being a stand-up comedian or a model. This does not mean that we can afford to overlook our presentation skills. In fact, some acting skills can be used to be a better communicator.
  - ○ Try to overcome stage fright and focus on communicating. There must be somebody out there interested in what you have to say.
  - ○ Avoid anything that would make you nervous when giving your presentation. One piece of advice is to remove all keys, coins, or other metal objects from your pockets so that you are not tempted to rattle them around – a truly irritating noise that we have all learned to hate.
  - ○ Put your cell phone (UK, mobile phone) and beeper on silent. The only thing more embarrassing than an attendee's cell phone interrupting your lecture is your own phone ringing in the middle of your talk.
  - ○ Eye contact: Remember to look at the audience and not only at your visual aid. Look around at the audience, not at the ceiling or floor.
  - ○ A big percentage of the impact that you will have on your audience depends on the way you look and behave. So, dress appropriately. But keep in mind that appropriate dressing means different things to different people. Also, it varies with the type of talk, the target audience, and the culture that they belong to. For example, if you do research on gene modified goods for agriculture, you may want to dress differently when you discuss your products with an audience of farmers than when you present them to financial advisors for potential investors in your company.

Useful Sentences to Comment on Images, Graphs, Tables,
Schematic Representations ...
- As you can see in the image on your right ...
- As you will see in the next table ...
- As we saw in the previous slide ...
- The next image shows ...
- The next image allows us to ...
- In the bottom left image we can see ...
- What do we have to look at here?
- What do we have to bear in mind with regard to this artifact?
- Notice how the lesion borders are ...
- Bear in mind that this image was obtained in less than 10 seconds ...
- Let's look at this schematic representation of the portal vein ...
- As you can see in this CT image ...
- Let us have a look at this schematic diagram of the portal system ...
- Looking at this table, you can see ...
- Having a look at this bar chart, we could conclude that ...
- To sum up, let's look at this diagram ...
- The image on your right ...
- The image at the top of the screen shows ...
- Let's turn to the next slide in which the lesion, after the administration of contrast material, is more conspicuous ...
- Figure 7 brings out the importance of ...
- I apologize that the faint bands in the Western blood *do not project well.* (When a subtle finding is difficult to see on a projected image, it is said that *it does not project well.*)
- On the left of the screen is a T2-weighted image at the level of the pons. On the right of the screen there is a *magnified view* of the abnormality.

3. **Say what you just said (i.e., Conclusions)**
   Summing up your "take-home" message should be pretty straightforward. If any points need reinforcing, this is the time to finish the presentation on a high note. Restate the main points that build your central message. Try to use different words to avoid repetition. This is not, however, the time to add any new information. The end of your talk also gives you an opportunity to acknowledge and thank not only the audience, which you must do, but also collaborators, the organizers of the meeting, and others. Below are a number of useful sentences to conclude your presentation.

Useful Sentences to Sum Up
- To sum up we can say that ...
- In summary, we have discussed ...
- To conclude ...

- Summing up, I would say that ...
- The take-home message of the talk is ...
- To put it in a nutshell ...
- To cut a long story short ...
- In short, ...
- To put it briefly ...
- Be that as it may, we have to bear in mind that ...
- If there is one point I hope you will take away from this presentation, it is that ...
- Thank you for your kind attention.
- Thank you all for sticking around until the very last talk of the session.
- Thank you all.
- Thank you for your attention. I would be happy to take any questions.
- Thank you for your time. I would be happy to address any questions.
- This is all we have time for, so thank you and have a good time in London.
- Let me finish my presentation by saying that ...
- We can say to conclude that ...
- Let me end by wishing you a pleasant stay in our city.
- I'd be happy to answer any questions you might have.
- I'd be happy to address your comments and questions.

The Dreaded Questions-and-Comments Section

Many beginners would not hesitate to deliver a free communication at an international congress if it weren't followed by a short section of questions.

This anecdote may illustrate the feelings of many non-native English-speaking biomedical scientists in their first presentations in English.

After a short free communication on the molecular mechanisms of synergism between stem cell factor and granulocyte-colony stimulating factor which had so far gone reasonably well for a beginner, I was waiting, like a rabbit staring at a snake, for the round of questions that inevitably followed my presentation. On the very verge of a mental breakdown, I listened to an American PI asking me a question I could barely understand. I told him: "Could you please repeat your question?" and he, obediently, repeated the question with exactly the same words and the same pace with which he had formulated it before. As I could not understand the question the second time, the chairman roughly translated it into a more international and easily understandable English and I answered it as best I could. This was the only question I was asked since the time was over and there was no room for any other comment.

Let us think about this anecdote in a positive way by dissecting it into the following points which will lead us to some recommendations.

1. Do not be discouraged. Nobody told you that beginnings were easy.
2. Questions and comments by native English speakers tend to be more difficult to understand than those made by non-native colleagues.
3. There are several types of interlocutors you must be aware of.
4. Do not complain if the interlocutor does exactly what you asked him/her for.
5. Chairmen can always help you.
6. Time is limited and you can take advantage of this fact.

These points lead to some recommendations:

1. I did not know at that point that the worst was still to come. I wasted the whole morning recreating the scene over and over. "How could I not have understood such an easy question? How could I have spoiled so many hours of research and study? I even thought that people recognized me as "the one who didn't understand a simple query …"

   Let us think for a moment how you performed the first time you did anything in your life, i.e., the first time you grabbed a tennis racquet or a golf club. In comparison to that, it was not that bad.

   As for the presentation itself, you need to be prepared for questions. That is correct. You can plan your spontaneity. You surely know the majority of possible loose ends in your presentation, the open questions, the target areas that are likely to be addressed by interlocutors. Do not leave it unprepared until the day of your talk. Work on it in advance. Think about the possible questions and prepare answers in English.

2. When the interlocutor who asks for the microphone is a non-native English speaker you can begin to feel better since you are going to talk to an equal with regard to language, to one who has spent a great number of hours fighting to learn a language other than his own. On the other hand, when you have to deal with a native English speaker there are two main types of interlocutors.

   Type A is a colleague who does not take advantage of being a native English speaker and reduces his normal rhythm of speech so you can understand the question and, therefore, convey to the audience whatever you have to say.

   Type B is a colleague who does not make any allowance for the difference between native and non-native English lecturers.

3. Types of interlocutors:
   - *Type 1*: Getting information. These interlocutors want to know a particular detail of your presentation, and are normally easy to handle by just answering the questions.
     - Make sure that you answer the question that was asked.
     - Rephrase the question for the audience and direct the answer to them although keeping the interlocutor involved.

   - *Type 2*: Show off. This interlocutor wants the audience to notice his sound knowledge of the subject which is being discussed. These are also quite easy to handle since they do not formulate questions as such but make a point of their own. Flattering always goes down well with this type. The replies tend to be shorter than the questions/comments and time, which runs in favor of the beginner provided he is not speaking, goes by, leaving no room for another dreaded question.

- *Type 3*: This is an interlocutor who strongly disagrees with your points. This is obviously the most difficult to handle for a beginner due to the scarcity of his idiomatic resources. In case of general disagreement make the interlocutor specify exactly what is it that he/she disagrees with. You are more likely to be able to defend specific pieces of data or results than more general abstract arguments. The best piece of advice is none other than that you must defend your points from a humble position and never get tangled up in a direct confrontation with your interlocutor.

4. If I had requested my interlocutor to ask his question again more slowly and in a different way so that I could understand it, he would have been morally obliged to do so. But beginners lack this kind of modesty and pretend to be better and know more than they actually are and do, which is, by definition, a mistake.
5. When you feel you need some help, ask the chairman to help you out.
6. It is, at worst, 1 minute of stress. Do not let such a short period of time prevent you from a potentially successful career in science.

Useful Sentences That May Help with Questions and Comments
Making Your Point
- Let me point out that signal intensity is paramount in order to differentiate …
- You must bear in mind that this evidence was obtained …
- If you look closely at this image, you will realize that …
- I want to draw your attention to the fact that …
- Don't forget the importance of …
- Before I move on to my next slide …
- In view of the upcoming publication of …
- Scientifically speaking …
- From a scientific point of view …
- As far as trackability is concerned …
- The bottom line of the subject is …

Giving Explanations
- To put it another way, contamination artifact was responsible for …
- Taking into consideration that the study was done under …
- In a bit more detail, you can notice that …
- This fact can be explained taking into account that …
- SNR (signal-to-noise ratio) in this 2D-gel is poor since the …
- Although the cell line eventually stops growing and differentiates, it provides an early phase of stable exponential expansion of …
- In short, you may need larger balloons in elderly patients.

- What I'm saying is that endometriosis is related to ectopic growth of endometrial tissue ...
- We have not been able to proceed with the animal experiments until ...
- We perform cell separation by cell sorting rather than by magnetic beads to better resemble subsequent experience in vivo with patients.

Answering Multiple Questions
- There are two different questions here.
- It seems there are three questions here.
- It is my understanding that there are two questions to be addressed here.
- With regard to your first question ...
- Regarding your second question ...
- As far as your first question is concerned ...
- Answering your first question, I should say that ...
- I'll begin with your second question.
- Let me address your last question first.
- I'll address your last question first and then the rest of them.
- Would you please repeat your second question?
- I didn't understand your first question. Would you repeat it?

Disagreeing
- With all due respect, I believe that there is no evidence of ...
- To the best of our knowledge, no article has been published on this topic.
- With all respect, I think that your point overlooks the main aspect of ...
- Yours is an interesting point of view, but I'm not sure of its ...
- I see it from a different point of view.
- With all respect, I don't go along with you on ...
- I think that the importance of ... cannot be denied.
- I strongly disagree with your comment on ...
- I disagree with your point.
- I don't see a valid argument for supporting such a comment.

Emphasizing a Point
- I do believe that ...
- I strongly agree with Dr. Ho's comments on ...
- It is of paramount importance ...
- It is a crucial fact that ...
- And this fact cannot be overlooked.
- I'd like to stress the importance of ...
- Don't underestimate the role of ...
- The use of DMSO in the control cases is of the utmost importance ...
- With regard to ..., you must always bear in mind that ...
- It is well known that ...

Incomprehension
- I'm not sure I understood your question …
- Sorry; I don't quite follow you.
- Would you repeat the question, please?
- Would you repeat the second part of your question, please?
- I'm afraid I still don't understand.
- Could you be a bit more specific with regard to …?
- What do you mean by …?
- Could you repeat your question? I couldn't hear you.
- Could you formulate your question in a different way?
- I'm not sure I understand your final question.

Playing for Time
- I am not sure I understood your question. Would you repeat it?
- I don't understand your question. Would you formulate it in a different way?
- That's a very interesting question …
- I wonder if you could be a bit more specific about …
- I'm glad you asked that question.
- Your question is of the utmost importance, but I'm afraid it is beyond the scope of our research …
- What aspect of the problem are you referring to by saying …

Evading an Issue
- I'm afraid I'm not really in a position to be able to address your question yet.
- We'll come back to that in a minute, if you don't mind.
- I don't think we have enough time to discuss your comments in depth.
- It would take extremely long time to answer that.
- I will address your question in my second talk, if you don't mind.
- At my institution, we do not have experience on …
- At our department, we do not perform …
- Perhaps we could return to that at the end of the session.
- We'll probably address your question in further papers on the subject.
- I have no experience of …

Technical Problems
- May I have another laser pointer?
- Does anyone in the audience have a pointer?
- Video images are not running properly. In the meantime I'd like to comment on …
- My microphone is not working properly. May I have it fixed?
- My microphone is not working properly. May I use yours?
- Can you hear me?
- Can the rows at the back hear me?
- Can you guys at the back see the screen?
- Can we turn off the lights please?

Practice, Practice, Practice

Yes, we know. The need for thorough planning and rehearsing of your presentation has been present in all sections of this chapter. Even for native English-speaking scientists, there is never too much planning and practice. Obviously, non-natives have to make an extra effort in this area. Practicing will improve your level of performance. More importantly, it will boost your self confidence, reduce your anticipated stress, and allow you to perform at a high level, close to your skill in your own language. So, practice, practice, practice.

Unit VIII   Chairing a Scientific Discussion

Chairing sessions at international meetings usually comes up when you have reached a certain level in your academic career. To reach this point many papers will have been submitted and many presentations will have been given, so the chances are that your level of biomedical English will be above that of the target audience of this manual.

Why, then, do we include a section on chairing a session?

We include it because contrary to what many of those who have never chaired a session in an international meeting may think, even an experienced chairperson with a reasonable level of English may face difficult, even embarrassing situations. Moreover, prior to chairing a larger scale session in an international meeting, you will have to learn to chair and bring together presentations from colleagues in smaller scale discussions, cooperative group meetings, or departmental retreats. Although the tone and level of formality may vary between these discussions, the skills and language resources you will require are very similar. Even in smaller meetings you will have to be able to introduce new colleagues, kick off and finish the discussion, manage questions, keep the schedule on time, or deal with technical problems. The sooner you start thinking about this type of scenario the more natural and fluent you will become for when the complexity and formality of the occasion increases.

For those who have never chaired a session, to be a chairman means, firstly, not having to prepare a presentation, and secondly, the use of simple sentences such as "thank you, Dr. Vida, for your interesting presentation" or "the next speaker will be Dr. Jones who comes from …". In our opinion, being a chairperson means much more than one who has never chaired them might think. To begin with, a chairperson must go over not one presentation but thoroughly review all the recently published material on the subject under discussion. On top of that, a chairperson must review all the abstracts and must have prepared questions just in case the audience has no questions or comments.

We have divided this chapter into four sections with practical suggestions and comments that will help you, as a non-native scientist, to successfully deal with various aspects of chairing a scientific discussion in English:

1. Usual chairperson's comments.
2. Should chairpersons ask questions?
3. What the chairperson should say when something is going wrong.
4. Specific scientific chairperson's comments.

R. Ribes et al., *English for Biomedical Scientists,*
DOI: 10.1007/978-3-540-77127-2_8, © Springer-Verlag Berlin Heidelberg 2009

Usual Chairperson's Comments

Everybody who has attended an international meeting is aware of the usual sentences the chairperson uses to introduce the session. Certain key expressions will provide you with a sense of fluency without which chairing a session would be troublesome. The good news is that if you know the key sentences and use them appropriately, chairing a session is easy. The bad news is that if, on the contrary, you do not know these expressions, a theoretically simple task may turn embarrassing. There is always a first time for everything, and if it is the first time you have been invited to chair a session, rehearse some of these sentences and you will feel quite comfortable. Accept this piece of advice: only "rehearsed spontaneity" looks spontaneous if you are a beginner.

Introducing the Session

We suggest the following useful comments for introducing the session:

- Good morning ladies and gentlemen. My name is Dr. Wu and I want to welcome you all to this workshop on animal models of graft-versus-host disease. My co-chair is Dr. Vick, from King's College.
- Good afternoon. The session on STAT Signaling and Cancer is about to start. Please take a seat and disconnect your cellular phones and any other electrical devices which could interfere with the oral presentations. We will listen to ten six-minute lectures with a two-minute period for questions and comments after each, and afterwards, provided we are still on time, we will have a last round of questions and comments from the audience.
- Good morning. We will proceed with the session on Oligodendrocyte Development. As many presentations have to be delivered I encourage the speakers to keep an eye on the time.

Introducing Speakers

We suggest the following useful comments for introducing speakers:

- Our first speaker is Dr. Ethel from Sutton, UK, who will present the paper: "Quality of life after reduced-intensity allogeneic transplantation."

The following speakers are introduced almost the same way with sentences such as:

- Our next lecturer is Dr. Adams. Dr. Adams comes from Brigham and Women's Hospital — Harvard Medical School. Her presentation today is entitled "Use of biomarkers to predict disease relapse after haematopoietic transplantation."
- Next is Dr. Shaw from Stanford University in California, presenting "MR approaches to molecular imaging."

- Dr. Olsen from UCSF is the next and last speaker. His presentation is: "Cardiac tissue regeneration using bone marrow derived stem cells."

Once the speakers finish their presentation, the chairperson is supposed to say something like:

- Thank you Dr. Olsen for your excellent presentation. Any questions or comments?

The chairperson usually comments on presentations, although sometimes they don ot:

- Thank you Dr. Olsen for your presentation. Are there any questions or comments from the audience?

There are some common adjectives (*nice, elegant, outstanding, excellent, interesting, clear, accurate* ...) and formulas that are usually used to describe presentations. These are illustrated in the following comments:

- Thanks Dr. Shaw for your accurate presentation. Does the audience have any comments?
- Thank you very much for your clear presentation on this always controversial topic. I would like to ask a question if I may (Although being the chairperson you are the one who gives permission, to ask the speaker is a usual formality.)
- I'd like to thank you for this excellent talk Dr. Olsen. Any questions from the audience?
- Thanks a lot for your very clear talk Dr. Ho. I wonder if the audience has got any questions.

Adjourning

We suggest the following useful comments for adjourning the session:

- I think we all are a bit tired so we'll have a short break.
- The session is adjourned until 4 p.m.
- We'll take a short break.
- We'll take a 30-minute break. Please fill out the evaluation forms.
- The session is adjourned until tomorrow morning. Enjoy your stay in Vienna.

Finishing the Session

We suggest the following useful comments for finishing the session:

- I'd like to thank all the speakers and the audience for your interesting presentations and comments. (I'll) see you all at the congress dinner and awards ceremony.

- The session is over. I want to thank all the participants for their contribution. (I'll) see you tomorrow morning. Remember to take your attendance certificates if you have not taken them already.
- We should finish up over here. We'll resume at 10:50.

Should Chairpersons Ask Questions?

In our opinion, chairpersons are supposed to ask questions especially at the beginning of the session when the audience does not usually make any comments at all. Warming-up the session is one of the chairperson's duties, and if nobody in the audience is in the mood to ask questions, the chairperson must invite the audience to participate:

- Are there any questions?

Nobody raises their hand:

- Well, I have got two questions for Dr. Adams. Are any of the biomarkers that you elegantly described likely to move from the research lab to clinical practice in our transplant patients? and second: What should be, in your opinion, their role in balance with clinical factors in diagnostic algorithms?

Once the session has been warmed-up, the chairperson should only ask questions or add comments as a tool to manage the timing of the session, so that, if as usual, the session is behind schedule, the chairperson is not required to participate unless strictly necessary.

The chairperson does not have to demonstrate to the audience his or her knowledge on the discussed topics by asking too many questions or making comments. The chairperson's knowledge of the subject is not in doubt since without it he or she would not have been selected to chair.

What the Chairperson Should Say When Something Is Going Wrong

Behind Schedule

Many lecturers, knowing beforehand they have a certain amount of time to deliver their presentations, try to talk a little bit more, stealing time from the questions/comments time and from later speakers. Chairpersons should cut short this tendency at the very first chance:

- Dr. Berlusconi, your time is almost over. You have got 30 seconds to finish your presentation.
- Dr. Ho, you are running out of time.

If the speaker does not finish his presentation on time, the chairperson may say:

- Dr. Berlusconi, I'm sorry but your time is over. We must proceed to the next presentation. Any questions, comments?

After introducing the next speaker, sentences such as the following will help you handle the session:

- Dr. Goyen, please keep an eye on the time, we are behind schedule.
- We are far from being ahead of schedule, so I remind all speakers you have six minutes to deliver your presentation.

Ahead of Schedule

Although unusual, sometimes there is some extra time and this is a good chance to ask the panelists a general question about their experience at their respective institutions:

- As we are a little bit ahead of schedule, I encourage the panelists and the audience to ask questions and offer comments.
- I have a question for the panelists: What percentage of the total number of CMRs at your institution are performed on children?

Technical Problems

Computer Not Working

We suggest the following comments:

- I am afraid there is a technical problem with the computer. In the meantime, I would like to make a comment about ...
- The computer is not working properly. While it is being fixed I encourage the panelists to offer their always interesting comments.

Lights Gone Out

We suggest the following comments:

- The lights have gone out. We'll take a hopefully short break until they are repaired.

- As you see, or indeed do not see at all, the lights have gone out. The hotel staff have told us it is going to be a matter of minutes so do not go too far; we'll resume as soon as possible.

Sound Gone Off

We suggest the following comments:

- Dr. Hoffman, we cannot hear you. There must be a problem with your microphone.
- Perhaps you could try this microphone?
- Please would you use the microphone, the rows at the back cannot hear you.

Lecturer Lacks Confidence

If the lecturer is speaking too quietly:

- Dr. Smith would you please speak up closer to your microphone? The audience does not seem to be able to hear you.
- Dr. Alvarez would you please speak up a bit? The people at the back cannot hear you.

If the lecturer is so nervous he/she cannot go on delivering the presentation:

- Dr. Higuchi, take your time. We can proceed to the next presentation, so whenever you feel OK and ready to deliver yours, it will be a pleasure to listen to it.

Specific Scientific Chairperson's Comments

Since chairpersons are supposed to fill in the gaps in the session, if a technical problem occurs, the chairperson must say something to entertain the audience in the meantime. This fact would not create any problem to a native English speaker but may be troublesome for a non-native English-speaking chairperson. In these situations there is always a helpful topic to be addressed "in the meantime," namely, the current situation of what is discussed in the session in the panelists' countries.

- Regarding the previous question on the role of genomics in this field, how applicable does the panel think it will be to daily clinical practice in the next 5 years?
- As for as the use of SPIO, what's the deal in Japan, Dr. Hashimoto?
- How is the current situation in Germany regarding repayment policies?

- May I ask how many of such studies you are performing yearly at your respective institutions?
- What's going on in the States in this topic, Dr. Olsen?

By opening a discussion on how things are going in different countries, the not-too-fluent chairperson shares the burden of filling in the gaps with the panelists. This trick rarely fails and once the technical problem is fixed the session can go on normally with nobody in the audience noticing the lack of fluency of the chairperson.

Besides the usual expressions that chairpersons have to be aware of, there are typical comments a scientific chairperson should be familiar with. These comments vary depending upon the scientific subspecialty of the chairperson and are, generally speaking, easy to deal with for even non-native English speakers. By way of example, let's review the following:

- Dr. Petit, would you please use the pointer to describe the confocal microscopy images that you are specifically referring to?
- Dr. Negroponte, how many control animals were used in each experiment?
- Did I understand correctly, Dr. Roberts, that the phosphorylation results that you just presented were obtained only in cell lines but not in primary tumor cells?
- Dr. Wilson, would you please point out the borders of the lesion so we can separate the tumor from the surrounding edema?
- Dr. Pons, I'm afraid that the video is not running properly. Could you try to fix it so we can see your excellent cell migration images?

UNIT IX

Unit IX   Curriculum Vitae, Cover Letters, and Other Professional Letters

Of all the non-native professionals targeted by the books in this series, biomedical scientists are the most likely to actually move to an English-speaking country to continue professional training and career development. Among the additional English needs that this professional move will require from you, the first task to tackle is writing your curriculum vitae (CV) and its cover letter.

If you are looking for a post in biomedical sciences, your CV is not only a brief written account of your personal, educational, and professional qualifications and experience. More importantly, your CV is your ticket to an interview. Whether the interview is for a new job opportunity, a scholarship, or for acceptance into graduate school, the way that your skills, education, experience, and professional goals are presented on your CV will be determinant to being successfully invited for an interview. In addition, your CV should always be accompanied by a cover letter. The purpose of the cover letter is not only to introduce yourself to the employer or evaluator and express your interest in the position that you are applying for. Your cover letter primarily gives you a brief opportunity to capture the recipient's attention and direct it towards information on your CV that is of particular value for the post.

This unit will give general guidance for biomedical scientists on how to write a CV and cover letter that stand out in English and, more importantly, for an English-speaking evaluator. General guidance on the design, sections, and lay out of CV and cover letters will be provided and explained with various examples and specific templates. Professional correspondence goes well beyond CVs and cover letters. Other professional letters that will be discussed in this unit include job acceptance and declination letters, resignation letters, and reference letters.

Professional Correspondence for Biomedical Scientists: General Tips

- Tailor your CV and, in particular, your cover letter specifically for each post. You are out to convince the employers that you have the qualities they require.

R. Ribes et al., *English for Biomedical Scientists*,
DOI: 10.1007/978-3-540-77127-2_9, © Springer-Verlag Berlin Heidelberg 2009

- Be concise and to the point. The evaluator will hardly have more than a few minutes to spend on your CV and cover letter. The cover letter should consist of one single page, and the CV should be no more than a few pages. This also means that the most recent and important information should be at the top of your CV.
- Use dynamic action verbs and an upbeat and positive language, but keep it under control and avoid exaggerated or inaccurate statements.
- Make sure there are no spelling, grammar, or punctuation mistakes. Employers will simply not tolerate any, regardless of being a native or non-native English speaker.

Curriculum Vitae

Your CV, or résumé in American English, is a short summary of your education, work experience, accomplishments, and other professional qualifications for the purpose of getting an interview when seeking a job. For most job applications, a prospective employer or principal investigator (PI) will often take a few minutes to read your CV and make a quick impersonal judgement of you. Therefore, you need to hook the reader by making a great impression. Writing a good CV will take time. There are no clear-cut rules governing the length and style of your CV. However, your CV should always be clear, concise, informative, and easy-to-read. Generally, it should only be a few pages in length. A longer or unfocused CV, while somewhat more acceptable in other cultures and languages, will only bore an English employer or admissions committee, and will surely find its way to the bin pretty quickly. The general tips on professional correspondence provided above must be used when preparing your CV.

All CVs should contain the following essential components:

- Personal information – This is placed at the start of the document, typically as a header. It should contain information such as your full name, current address, e-mail address, home phone number, and cellular number. Your name should be the first text on the CV.
- Education information – This is a vital section on your CV. List your education in reverse chronological order. Keep in mind that once you have a degree and some work experience, anything less than a Bachelor's degree can be left out (such as primary and secondary education).
- Training courses – List any work-related training courses which you have attended.
- Work experience – This is an essential element. Your work experience should be listed in reverse chronological order, starting with the most recent job and moving backwards. Add details such as employer, position, dates (start and finishing), and duties.

- Major achievements – Here you can add awards, scholarships, fellowships, prizes and grants.
- Publications – This section typically appears near the end of a CV. If you have numerous publications then select the most important and relevant papers. You can state that a full list is available upon request.

Things NOT to include in your CV:

- A picture of yourself (unless you're applying for a modeling or acting position).
- Personal details not relevant to the job such as date of birth, height, weight, gender, sexual orientation, religion, race, marital status, whether or not you have children, or even your hobbies. You should not be judged based on these types of personal details.
- Writing in the first person. Do not begin sentences with the word 'I' or 'me.' Replace these pronouns with action verbs such as Evaluated, Assessed, Established, Maintained, Researched, Developed, Coordinated.
- Images, tables, text boxes.
- Incorrect details or lies. These will often be discovered by the employer when he/she does a reference or background check.
- Past, current, and expected salary.
- Past failures or health problems.
- Reasons for leaving a job.
- List of references. This is a waste of valuable space. Do not include them until asked.
- Spelling mistakes and grammatical errors.
- Making it too fancy and complicated by using colorful inks or fancy fonts.

Once you're done writing your CV, you should always seek feedback. Ask your trusted colleagues and friends to look it over and give you some advice.

Here is an example of a CV:

Alex Mackenzie
29 Queen Street West
Toronto, ON M5V 2Z5
(416) 338-6320

EDUCATION

Ph.D. IN Developmental Biology   **To be completed in 2008**
University of Toronto   **Toronto, ON, CA**
"The role of platelet-derived growth factor receptor α in mouse
development", supervised by Drs. John Abbott and Alan Davis.

Harvard University
  Introduction to Immunology
  Introduction to Cancer Biology

HONORS B.Sc. IN BIOLOGY   **Completed 1999**
McGill University   **Montreal, QC, CA**
  Major in Biology, minor in Chemistry with relevant courses including
  Microbiology, Molecular & Cellular Biology, Biochemistry, Molecular Genet-
  ics, Bacterial Genetics, and Virology.

RESEARCH EXPERIENCE

RESEARCH ASSISTANT   **June 2002-April 2004**
University of Cambridge   **Cambridge, UK**

- gained extensive knowledge of bacterial genetic techniques, including the
  ligation of gene clones, plasmid extraction, DNA digestion with restriction
  enzymes, Northern and Southern blot transfers, the preparation of competent
  bacteria and aseptic technique
- performed library screening
- participated in the animal research section of the laboratory by the
  generation, characterization and utilization of transgenic mouse lines
- trained in the isolation, modification and purification of P1 derived
  Artificial Chromosomes (PACs) for the generation of transgenic mice
- expertise in pronuclear DNA microinjection in mouse embryos and
  embryo transfer
- maintained several mice colonies
- performed sample preparation and tissue staining/labeling, such as Immunohistochemistry, In Situ Hybridization, LacZ, BrdU, Sudan Black
- experienced in light, fluorescence and confocal microscopy
- served as a liaison between the laboratory and the Institute's Genetic
  Modification Safety Officer to ensure proper and valid assessments have been
  made on the risks to human health and safety and to the environment

RESEARCH TECHNICIAN   July 1998-2000
Sr. Research Technician   August 2000-April 2002
Harvard University   Boston, MA, USA

- conducted neuro-oncology experiments: specifically with regards to growth factors, receptors and signalling pathways that are relevant in the pathogenesis of central and peripheral nerve tumours
- generated, purified, characterized and utilized activated state specific phosphopeptide antibodies to receptor tyrosine kinases
- conducted in vivo studies on potential chemotherapeutic drug STI571
- performed culture, maintenance, and generation of protein extracts from several different cell lines
- performed Western blot analysis
- examined the differentiation potential of primary stem cells using retroviral and adenoviral ectopic expression systems
- performed immunohistochemistry/immunocytochemistry
- performed RNA purification & Northern blot analysis
- performed DNA purification & PCR analysis
- prepared and transformed competent cells
- assisted with the general, common laboratory work of making solutions, autoclaving, and similar duties

PUBLICATIONS

Selected significant publications are listed below. Full list is available upon request.

MacKenzie, A., Abbott, J. and Macdonald, J.A. (2008) "Identification and characterization of the mouse PDGFRα gene", Nature 800, 454-466.

MacKenzie, A., Laurier, W., Thompson, J. and Macdonald, J.A. (2007) "PDGFRalpha gene mutation and protein expression in glioma brain tumors", Oncology 89, 91-97.

Stronzo, S., Bennett, R.B., MacKenzie, A., Chang, L., Wang, F. and Miller, A. (2004) "PAC modification and generation of Sox10-Cre transgenic mice", Genesis 64, 335-346.

AWARDS

Canadian Graduate Scholarship (CGS) Award 2005
Undergraduate Student Research Award (USRA) 1998

REFERENCES AVAILABLE UPON REQUEST

COVER LETTER

A cover letter, also called a covering letter, is a document sent with your résumé or curriculum vitae to provide the potential employer with additional information. The cover letter is just as important as the résumé because it is normally read first and if the prospective employer or principal investigator is not impressed with it, both the cover letter and résumé will be thrown in the trash. The main purpose of a cover letter is to get the employer or PI to read your résumé.

Cover letters should be no longer than one typed page. How do you keep it short and still deliver enough information to catch the reader's attention? We suggest you to write your cover letter based on the following structure:

- Address your cover letter to a specific person by name and title (e.g. Dear Dr. XXX) and end it with "Sincerely." Alternatively, if you are unable to get the name then use "Dear Sir or Madam" for the salutation, and end it with "Yours faithfully."
- A first paragraph to introduce yourself and to state why you are writing.
- A second paragraph to briefly describe your professional and academic qualifications that are relevant to the job position.
- A third paragraph to emphasize what you can do for the laboratory should also state how your career objectives fit the job objectives.
- A final paragraph to conclude your letter by reconfirming your interest in the job, indicate that you are available for an interview, express your willingness to provide additional information, and thank the reader for their time and consideration.

Cover letters generally fall into three major types: advertised response cover letters, speculative cover letters, and referral cover letters.

- ***Advertised response cover letters*** are the easiest to write of the three types of cover letters. This type of letter is written in response to an advertised job opening. Use the information on the job advertisement to help you write the cover letter. Respond to each and every required skill, education, and experience listed in the job advertisement, and provide evidence for this.
- ***Speculative cover letters*** are letters regarding possible job opportunities written to potential employers or PIs who have not advertised or published job openings. Human resources and PIs are often inundated with many of these on a monthly basis. So, it is important you make a great impression. You also need to give the person reading your cover letter a compelling reason to continue reading it. Even though you are not applying for an advertised position, you must demonstrate your knowledge of, and interest in, the laboratory you

are writing to. You also need to demonstrate to the potential employer why they would want you in their laboratory. Sell yourself!

- *Referral cover letters* are letters sent to potential employers that you came to know through your friends or colleagues. Never underestimate the power of networking. Employers often prefer to hire someone who is known to at least one colleague. Referral cover letters are very similar to speculative cover letters, the main difference being that a referral cover letter should mention the individual who referred you to the job, employer, or laboratory.

In this unit we provide you with a few examples of cover letters. The details are, of course, fictitious. These letters should only be used as a guide since your cover letter should illustrate your own skills and education, and should be customized to meet the needs of the potential employer and the type of post that you are applying for.

Example 1

This is a sample cover letter for a position as a research assistant at an academic institution, and it is written in response to a publicized job listing.

28 Woodstock Road
Oxford, England
OX2 6HB

August 2, 2008

Human Resources
McMaster University Medical Centre
Hamilton, ON, Canada

Dear Sir or Madam:

Please consider my application for the Research Assistant position, Job Opening Number 94563. I am particularly interested in this position, which relates strongly to my eight years of experience as a research assistant in several world-class universities.

I am originally from France, where I received a four year degree in Biological Sciences with a minor in Chemistry from École Normale Superieure de Paris in 2000. Subsequently, I moved to Boston (Massachusetts), where I gained valuable experience in neurodevelopmental biology while working as a Research Technician in the laboratory of Professor Charles Paulines at Harvard Medical School. Since July 2004, I have been working as a Research Assistant in the neurodevelopmental genetics laboratory of Professor William Smith at Oxford University. My eight year work experience has provided me with a solid foundation for research. I believe that this experience would be of value for the position advertised.

Thank you for your consideration of my application. My résumé is enclosed for your perusal. Please contact me should you require any further information.

Yours faithfully,

Amélie Dubois

Example 2

Here is an example of a speculative cover letter for an unadvertised postdoctoral position. In this case, always address the letter to a specific person by name and title.

Via dei Capocci 203
00184 Rome, Italy

July 10, 2008

Domenico I. Sirolli, PhD
Department of Neuroscience
Stanford University
300 Pasteur Drive
Stanford, CA, USA

Dear Dr. Sirolli,

I am writing this letter to inquire about the possibility of obtaining a Postdoctoral position within your research group. I have enclosed a copy of my CV for your consideration.

I am currently a PhD student in the Department of Biomedical Sciences at La Sapienza University in Rome, expecting to complete my degree requirements in September 2008. My PhD thesis project is under the guidance and supervision of Professor Tim Horttons. In my thesis project, I looked at the ability of transplanted neural stem cells containing a reporter gene to rescue injured tissue after ischemic injury in mice. I also characterised the effects of ischemic injury on the endogenous population of stem cells in the subventricular zone and found these cells are activated; which then lead me to determine the molecular signals that are responsible for their activation.

My laboratory skills involved generating constructs and transgenic mice and analysing in the migration of both the endogenous and transplanted stem cell by in situ hybridization and immunohistochemistry. I believe that this profile may fit well with the research interests and focus of your group.

I would be grateful if you would consider me for any current or future vacancies that might arise with your laboratory.

Sincerely,

Marisa Di Prata

Example 3

A referral letter is very similar to a speculative cover letter; the only main difference is that you need to include the name of the person who referred you to the laboratory in the first paragraph. Let's take the previous example and adapt it accordingly.

Via dei Capocci 203
00184 Rome, Italy

July 10, 2008

Domenico I. Sirolli, PhD
Department of Neuroscience
Stanford University
300 Pasteur Drive
Stanford, CA, USA

Dear Dr. Sirolli,

I am writing this letter **following the advice of Dr Tim Horttons, my thesis supervisor**, to inquire about the possibility of obtaining a Postdoctoral position within your research group. I enclosed a copy of my CV for your consideration.

I am currently a PhD student **in Dr Horttons' group** in the Department of Biomedical Sciences at La Sapienza University in Rome, expecting to complete my degree requirements in September 2008. My PhD thesis project is under the guidance and supervision of Professor Tim Horttons. In my thesis project, I looked at the ability of transplanted neural stem cells containing a reporter gene to rescue injured tissue after ischemic injury in mice. I also characterised the effects of ischemic injury on the endogenous population of stem cells in the subventricular zone and found these cells are activated; which then lead me to determine the molecular signals that are responsible for their activation.

My laboratory skills involved generating constructs and transgenic mice and analysing the migration of both the endogenous and transplanted stem cell by in situ hybridistion and immunohistochemistry. I believe that this profile may fit well with the research interests and focus of your group.

I would be grateful if you would consider me for any current or future vacancies that might arise with your laboratory.

Sincerely,

Marisa Di Prata

Other Professional Letters

Job Acceptance Letter

Many job offers and subsequent acceptances of an offer are generally made over the phone. However, it is a good idea to confirm your acceptance in writing. The contents of this letter should include your appreciation for the offer and pre-determined employment conditions such as salary, start date, and benefits. A job acceptance letter ensures that you and your employer have a common understanding about the terms of your employment.

550 Holimont Crt
Hamilton, ON
L9C 0B1

August 25, 2008

Adelia I. Frade, PhD
Department of Biomedical Sciences
McMaster University Medical Centre
1200 Main Street West
Hamilton, ON L8N 3Z5

Dear Dr. Frade,

I am delighted to accept your offer as a Research Assistant in your laboratory. I have been very impressed with everyone whom I have met in your group during my interview and I look forward to joining your lab.

As we agreed, my starting date will be September 25 to enable me to finish my current research project. I understand that my annual salary will be $35,000 and I will receive three weeks of annual paid vacation.

If there is any further information I need prior to my start date, I can be reached at (905) 5746689. I am looking forward to working with you and your research team.

Thank you again for this opportunity.

Sincerely,

Jane Wilson

Declination Letter

It is proper business etiquette and a matter of courtesy to acknowledge an offer that you are rejecting. Declination letters are the formal way to do this. In this type of letter you should graciously decline the offer, briefly explain the reason for your declination, and thank the individual for the offer.

550 Holimont Crt
Hamilton, ON
L9C 0B1

August 25, 2008

Adelia I. Frade, PhD
Department of Biomedical Sciences
McMaster University Medical Centre
1200 Main Street West
Hamilton, ON L8N 3Z5

Dear Dr. Frade,

Thank you very much for offering me the position of Research Assistant in your laboratory.

After considerable thought, I have decided to decline your offer and accept another job offer. Though this was a difficult decision, I believe the other job offer closely matches my current career goals and interests.

Thank you very much for the time and consideration that you have given me. I wish you luck in your search for an appropriate candidate.

Sincerely,

Jane Wilson

Resignation Letter

A resignation letter is a formal letter stating your intention to quit your position. This type of letter must be short, simple, and to the point. The tone of the letter should be positive and professional, even if you didn't like your job or are leaving under bad circumstances. Do not use a resignation letter as a way to complain about your job or criticize your boss or co-workers. Remember that you may want a reference from them in the future.

At a minimum, your letter should contain:

- Last expected day of employment.
- Very brief reason for your resignation.
- Expression of thanks for the opportunity to work in his/her laboratory.

550 Holimont Crt
Hamilton, ON
L9C 0B1

July 20, 2008

Adelia I. Frade, PhD
Department of Biomedical Sciences
McMaster University Medical Centre
1200 Main Street West
Hamilton, ON L8N 3Z5

Dear Dr. Frade,

Please accept this letter as formal notice of my resignation from the position of Research Assistant, with effect from August 20. I hope that a month notice will give you enough time to find a suitable replacement.

I have decided to move on and have accepted a new position elsewhere, which I believe will enable me to further my career.

It has been a pleasure working for you and I wish you the very best for the future.

Yours sincerely,

Jane Wilson

Reference Letter

A reference letter, also known as a recommendation letter, is a formal letter used to introduce a job applicant and give personal assurance for his/her integrity, character, and ability. Most reference letters are written by former employers. If one of your trainees or colleagues is planning to move to an English-speaking lab, you are very likely to be asked to write a reference letter for him/her. It goes without saying that you must be honest in your assessment of the applicant. It is best to decline to write a reference letter if you cannot give a good recommendation.

While writing a reference letter there are certain points, listed below, that you should keep in mind:

- Open the letter with a formal business greeting such as "Dear XXX," "Dear Sir or Madam," or "To whom it may concern."
- State that you recommend the candidate: "It is with great pleasure that I write this recommendation for John A. Smith."
- Give a very brief background of how you know the applicant and how long you have known him/her. You can include dates of employment. You should also introduce yourself by stating your position and title.
- Describe the applicant's strengths, skills, and qualifications. Focus on skills and qualities relevant to the job the applicant is seeking.
- Include personal qualities of the applicant.
- Use positive powerful adjectives such as honest, excellent, superior, efficient, dependable, creative, reliable, observant, assertive.
- Avoid weak adjectives such as nice, good, fair, OK.
- Make the ending of your letter strong: "I am confident that he/she will become an important asset to your research team and recommend him/her without reservations."
- Offer to provide more information and list your own contact details: "I am happy to provide further information if required."
- Keep the letter to one page in length.

Harvard Medical School
25 Shattuck Street
Boston, MA 02115

August 10, 2008

Adelia I. Frade, PhD
Department of Biomedical Sciences
McMaster University Medical Centre
1200 Main Street West
Hamilton, ON L8N 3Z5

Dear Dr. Adelia Frade,

It is with great pleasure that I write this recommendation for Dr. John A. Smith. I have known Dr. Smith for five years, both as his employer at Harvard Medical School from 2000 through 2003, and as a professional colleague.

Dr. Smith is a talented young scientist on an upward path of career growth. During his time in my laboratory, he performed at a very high level. He showed highly developed scientific skills, sound knowledge of multiple areas in Developmental Biology, and had an excellent command of the literature. He combines these talents with a very strong work ethic to make him particularly productive. This is reflected in the fact that he has published five scientific papers in prestigious scientific journals in just three years.

Beyond his scientific skills, Dr. Smith has all the interpersonal traits that one looks for in a colleague. Dr. Smith is friendly, interactive, and conscientious. Moreover, he has a proficient degree of maturity and independence for his young age.

I am confident that Dr. Smith will become a valued member of your laboratory. I recommend him without reservation. If I may provide you with any further information in your consideration of Dr. Smith, please feel free to contact me.

Sincerely,

Tina Alongi, PhD
Professor of Biology
Harvard Medical School
(617) 432-1550 Office
(617) 432-3307 (Fax)
t.alongi@hms.harvard.edu

UNIT X

Unit X   Getting Ready for a Job Interview in English

Unit IX has just shown you how to write a CV and cover letter that can make your qualifications and experience look competitive for a job application. So, if you got invited for an interview: congratulations, you've successfully passed the first round! The job, however, is far from over. If you want to finish it and get an offer for the position that you are applying for, you will have to confirm that good initial impression from your résumé in a job interview. Even more, as a non-native English-speaking applicant, you will have to confirm that good first impression in an interview held in a language that is not your own.

Self-confidence is your most effective quality in a job interview. You will have to look inside yourself, remember who you are, what you have done so far, why you are applying to that particular post, and identify everything that you have to offer to the potential employer. And then, you will have to sell it. In a job interview, the employers expect you to provide them with all the additional information that they couldn't get from your résumé to help them make a fully informed decision about the right candidate for the post. And there is no other way to do so than by talking about your own assets and strengths. Presenting yourself in a job interview in a negative way that apologizes for the things you haven't done rather than making a strong case for the things you have done is not a sign of honesty. It is a sign of plain stupidity. The likely outcome of such an approach is that the job will go to someone else. And rightly so, we'd dare to add. Some people, however, would rather play themselves down than making the effort to present an accurate and exciting image of themselves. If you are one of them, you may want to skip this unit. But if you value yourself and are willing to make the effort to defend your value in a job interview in English, you will find this unit particularly useful. Here, we will provide you with specific information and advice to successfully face this challenge. We'll go through your preparation up to the day of the interview, as well as the interview itself, and give some notes on what to do the day after.

You Are More Than Your Level of English

It is pretty obvious that when applying for a job in biomedical sciences in an English-speaking lab, the language is just a means to an end (i.e., effective communication) and not the focus of either your job or job interview. Even

R. Ribes et al., *English for Biomedical Scientists*,
DOI: 10.1007/978-3-540-77127-2_10, © Springer-Verlag Berlin Heidelberg 2009

so, many non-native English-speaking candidates put all their attention on the possible language-barrier difficulty when facing a job interview in English. We understand that you may neither be at your best in English, nor feel as convincing as you may be in your own language. For this reason, this chapter will take you through the various steps of a job interview in English and provide you with examples and model questions and answers to get you ready for your interview. These tools will help you refocus away from the language itself and back on professional issues that are more likely to be decisive in the hiring decision. Practising is no doubt required for all applicants, and it is even more critical for non-native speakers. But do not get overstressed, the majority of English-speaking employers and PIs do indeed appreciate and value the additional effort that international scientists have to make in order to settle in an English-speaking environment. And that appreciation works to your advantage.

You Are More Than Your Résumé

Even if your CV was good at getting you an interview, you have got much more to offer in that interview that what's on your CV. Moreover, you have got to offer much more in that interview that what's on your CV. Employers and PIs are busy people. If all that they were interested in could be read in a résumé, they would not bother interviewing anybody. They would just appoint whoever handed in the best CV. But they don't. So, what is it that they want? What will they be expecting from you in your interview?

Let's take a look at the following job advertisement for a minute:

August 1st, 2008

Postdoctoral Position in Neurodevelopmental Biology, Seattle, Washington

Description:
Postdoctoral position available for NSF funded project to study the molecular basis of brain development in Dr. George Chen's laboratory at the University of Washington in Seattle. Current focus of research is on transcription factors as key regulators of development, in particular TXUK and SOX families that regulate tissue differentiation. Funding is available for 2 years beginning April 1st, 2009.

Requirements:
PhD in Neurosciences, molecular, cellular, developmental biology or related field. Basic cellular and molecular biology and microscopy skills required. Ability to perform in situ hybridizations, cloning and transgenic techniques desired. Highly motivated, mature and responsible scientist committed to working in a competitive academic environment sought.

Applications:
Review of applications will begin immediately and continue until the position has been filled. Please send CV, cover letter and 3 reference contacts to: George Chen, Department of Biology, University of Washington, Seattle WA 98195. E-mail: george_chen@u.washington.edu

Let's imagine that you sent in your application and you have been short-listed to be interviewed. There will be two other candidates for the post.

What are the chances that your credentials will be significantly different from the other candidates'?

Very small, we should think. People without a PhD in the field or lacking the type of experience requested would not have made it through the cut into the interview. People with far greater experience would be unlikely to apply for a postdoctoral position funded by a research project for two years with potential caveats for someone more senior, such as unclear expectations for the longer term.

So, if the other candidates come in with basically comparable résumés, the interview is your real chance to show that you are the best candidate beyond what's on your résumé; your chance to show that you are indeed the best fit for the job. How do you do that?

Find Out About the Employer and Interviewers

Before going to a job interview you must learn about your potential employer and interviewers. You must know about their research interests and be aware of their published work, in particular recent work. And beyond what you may find in the scientific literature, you should find out additional useful information about them. Check the web page of the company or university. Check their newsletters and brochures, their annual activity reports, or at the very least just go ahead and google them!

Knowing about your potential employer is also useful for you in that you can better judge whether the job is right for you or not. When you decide that the job is good for you, you must be able to explain your reasons to the employer, to explain them in English, and to support those reasons on a good understanding of the company and what the post entails. This understanding can only come from thorough research. You must prepare to be able to tell the interviewers about your interest in the post, and as long as you have prepared it well, we think that you may want to tell them whether or not they ask you about it.

Researching your potential employer and interviewers will also provide you with useful information to try and put yourself in their position. Put yourself in the interviewers' shoes and think of the way they are going to be looking at you from the other side of the table. What is it that they are looking for? What are the current areas of interest and future directions that they seem to be pointing at? Also, you should project yourself into the job. Try and see yourself in the post and figure out which of your current skills they may lack, and which you could bring into the job and the team.

You Must Prepare for Your Interview

Preparation is the key to a smooth interview process for any candidate. But if you are being interviewed in a foreign language, preparation is even more critical. You do not want to take the chance of improvising here. In addition, having prepared thoroughly for your interview will reduce your nervousness and make you more confident and fluent.

At the end of the day, a job interview is an interactive performance with the main objective of selling yourself as the ideal candidate for the post. We have already gone through several aspects of presenting in English in unit VII, and would like to go back to that discussion and apply it to the job interview setting. As we put it before, being a good researcher or a competent scientist is not the same thing as being a stand-up comedian, an actor or a model. Your only goal is communicating with the interviewers. Keep in mind that the members of an interview panel for a research post are not professional interviewers. They are scientists and academics and their real goal is to make sure they hire the candidate that is going to fit best in the group, they are going to be happy supervising, and that is most likely to be productive. In a nutshell, they are looking for the candidate that they like (professionally) the best. So, you must prepare yourself to make them like you the best, and you cannot afford to overlook the way that you present yourself:

- Overcome your fears: fear of failure in obtaining the job, fear of making a fool of yourself with the language barrier, failure of rejection … and focus on communicating. You will never know how well you can do if you do not try. Give yourself and the employers some credit. If the employers called you in to find out more about your potential in an interview, they must be interested in what you have to say. In a way, you do belong there already.
- Dress appropriately. A professional appearance is a good way to let the employer know that you know what is appropriate in the workplace. And it doesn't require any conversational effort. Keep in mind that appropriate dressing means different things for different people. Also, it varies with the type of job, the level of seniority, and the culture that they belong to. In case of doubt, our advice would be to lean more towards a conservative style, more so than you would normally follow for your everyday hands-on lab work. At the end of the day, you will be judged by your professional image. If you are still unsure about the way to dress, you may want to try accessing photos of the people in the lab from the center's website biographical sketches, the net, or even try and pay an undercover visit to the university or centre to look at it firsthand. Once you make a decision about your interview attire, you must

try it on. Make sure that it fits and that you feel comfortable with it. Go out on the street or to your current job wearing it and see what feed-back you get from other people. You may feel surprised by the positive effect of making that little effort. Looking good and feeling good about the way you look for your job interview will also increase your confidence and will make you perform better on the day.

- Behave appropriately. The main goal of your physical communication with the interviewers is to help create a positive atmosphere for communication. You have to keep your body language open and relaxed, and show that you listen and that you focus on your interaction with them. Keeping eye contact during the discussion is an obvious part of such an open body language. But do not put all your attention on a long list of physical do's and don'ts (e.g., how to sit on the chair, how to use your hands …), that may end up making you behave unnaturally and too self-consciously. Try to keep the focus on communicating a positive message, as well as your strengths and value for the post. It should go without saying that you must avoid anything that would make you or the interviewers uncomfortable or nervous during the interview. Put your cell phone (*UK* mobile phone) and beeper on silent. The only thing more embarrassing and annoying than an interviewer's cell phone interrupting the interview is your own phone ringing in the middle of your interview. One additional piece of advice is to remove all keys, coins, or other metal objects from your pockets so that you are not tempted to rattle them around.
- Be prepared to answer questions. That is correct: spontaneity in a foreign language must be prepared for. Most questions do not just happen randomly. They can and must be predicted. You should be able to identify the majority of potential loose ends in your résumé, as well as the employer's areas of interest from where open questions may come. At the end of the unit we will provide you with additional model questions to practice with. Do not leave questions and answers unprepared until the day of the interview. Work on them in advance and prepare your answers directly in English. Write them down and rehearse them. You'll be happy you did it right at the very second that you hear the interviewer formulating a question that you have prepared for. You won't only have an answer in English ready, but your confidence will multiply right on the spot and your answer will be more convincing.
- Be prepared to ask questions. The most common, predictable, and critical question in a job interview is the last one:

*"Well, Ms Wu. We would like to thank you for making the time to come down to this interview and for answering our questions. We still have time before we finish, and we would like to know: **do you have any questions for us?**"*

Some interviewees would actually wrongly believe that at this point their interview job is nearly finished. Even more in the case of non-native interviewees speaking in English, the easiest way out of this challenge would appear to be shrugging their shoulders and not asking any questions to finish as soon as possible. Without a doubt, this would be an UNFORGIVABLE MISTAKE. Your questions to the interviewers are the most decisive part of your job interview. They are not an option. You must ask questions. Just put yourself in the interviewers' shoes. They are very busy people; they have kindly called you in to get to know you better and to find out more about your suitability for the post; a post that they have an obvious interest in and would like to recruit the best candidate for. And you don't have either the intelligence or the professional courtesy to formulate a few meaningful questions (?). You might as well have arrived at the interview late, with a sloppy appearance, and checked text messages on your cell phone halfway through. The outcome is going to be just as bad. Not asking any questions equals, in the interviewers minds, one or several of the following: you are too uninterested in the job to make the effort to inquire any further; you are too easily intimidated to interact proactively with your potential employer; you are too stupid to conclude anything out of 10, 20 or 30 minutes of conversation with them; or you are too disrespectful to really grab the opportunity they are giving you to get the post. In any case, it will surely kill any chances to be offered the post that you may have created up to that point. So, prepare several meaningful questions for the interviewers. Even if some of them were possibly addressed earlier during the interview (those you obviously would not ask again at the end), you will still have a few relevant questions to discuss with the panel at the end. We will provide you with some examples of such questions at the end of the unit. Make sure you do prepare them in advance directly in English, write them down, and rehearse them.

Practice, Practice, Practice...

Yes, we know. The need for thorough planning and rehearsing of your presentation has been present in other sections of this unit. Even for native English-speaking candidates undergoing a job interview, there is never too much planning and practice. Obviously, non-natives have to make an extra effort. Practicing will improve your level of performance. More importantly, it will boost your self-confidence, reduce your anticipated stress, and allow you to perform at a high level, close to your skill in your own language. So, practice, practice, practice...

How do you practice? We recommend you to put all the information you have collected in writing: your skills, your training, your strengths, your employer's information, and a list of questions and answers, all in English. Once you have all that material ready you will have to practice with it. And when we say practice, we mean practice for real; as real as you can get it. Practice on your own at first, but practice for your real job interview with a real mock interview. The same way that after watching the downhill skiing championships on the sports channel, and after talking to skier friends, you had better take a practical skiing course before going on the slopes on your own, once you've done your research and prepared for your interview, you have to do a real training session. This is a mock interview. And for a real mock interview, you need a real mock interviewer. Our advice would be that you ask your English teacher to mock interview you.

Alternatively, you may want to choose a friend or colleague with a good level of English. In any case, you must work seriously on this final exercise, and make it as real as you can. Otherwise, you won't get much out of it. And when we say real, we mean that you should wear the same clothes that you're planning to wear to the real interview, you should allocate the same time that you will be given for the real interview, and you will have to set it up as a real interview: set up a particular place for it, an agreed time, make sure that you introduce yourself to the interviewer upon arrival, and act as you would do in the real interview. Your mock interviewer will have to be given your CV, and the list of questions that you want to rehearse ahead of time, and you will have to make him/her aware that you want the mock interview to be carried out in as realistic a way as possible. This is the time to act your interviewee role at your best. So, warm up, get ready and enjoy the experience! Do you think that this may be stressful or silly? Well, on the real interview day you'll be happy that you made the effort.

What Else Should You do on the Day of the Interview?

The only thing that kept your thorough preparation and your mock inspection from being a real rehearsal is that it didn't take place on the real set. On the day of the job interview you must give yourself plenty of time to get ready and arrive on the set of the interview well ahead of time. Make sure that you have a look around the interview facilities, make yourself familiar with the environment, and make yourself feel comfortable there. Also make sure that you look good and feel good about the way you look for your interview. In addition, try to remember all the positive qualities that you have revised about yourself, and focus on the added value that you can bring to the advertised job. Keep your one or two main strengths in your mind and try to feel good about the expectations of sharing those with the interviewers. Remind yourself of all the work you have done to prepare for the interview, and of how you have covered the majority of topics, questions, and answers that you are likely to have to deal with.

The chances are that despite your preparation you'll be a little nervous on the day of your interview. That is not only normal, but probably good as well. Normal people get nervous in situations of this kind. And a little nervousness will give you the energy and drive to make the effort in the interview. It makes you more alert, possibly smarter. You are ready to go. So, enjoy the ride, and the interview rush.

The Day After: What to do After Your Interview?

The first thing you should do after you are done with the interview is treating yourself to something special you know you will enjoy. You've gone all the way through with your interview in English. Congratulations! In the worst case scenario, you've learned a lot and made yourself more experienced and competitive. But, is there anything else you can do the day after your interview?

Once you have cooled down and given yourself a treat, the day after the interview is the time to reflect on your performance in the real job interview experience. The quality of your performance does not necessarily associate with getting the job. Employers may be looking for a different profile or type of person. If that was the case, it's possibly not such a bad thing for you to realize, even at this later stage, that the job was not right for you. Don't take it personally though if the outcome is not positive. Remember that to some extent it was just a performance, and that you are taking a good deal of experience from it with you. The key consideration here is identifying what you would do the same or differently in the next interview.

On the other hand, if the outcome of the interview is not available immediately, you may certainly want to contact the employer and send a follow-up thank you letter. At the very least, you can thank them for their time and the opportunity to meet them. We include an example of such a type of letter below:

550 Holimont Crt
Hamilton, ON
L9C 0B1

August 7, 2008

Adelia I. Frade, PhD
Department of Biomedical Sciences
McMaster University Medical Centre
1200 Main Street West
Hamilton, ON L8N 3Z5

Dear Dr. Frade,

I would like to express my sincere gratitude for meeting with me on Monday, August 6. I enjoyed learning more about your research and the position you described. I left with the strong conviction that I will fit in beautifully as a member of your research team. And I would also like to reiterate my strong interest in the position you have available.

I look forward, Dr. Frade, to hearing from you concerning your hiring decision. Again, thank you for your time and consideration.

Sincerely,

Adalgisa Fratelli

Questions and Answers

Questions you have to ask yourself in preparation for the interview

What are the primary objectives of the post? Why am I interested in this job?	*This should be the main initial focus of your research of the company and the post. You must be able to explain reasons of your interest in the job to your employer, to explain them in English, and to support those reasons on a good understanding of the company and what the post entails. As we mentioned above, you should probably tell them why you are interested in the post whether or not they ask you about it, and as long as you have prepared this questions well.*
How does my training fit with the requirements of the post?	*You should identify parts of your training that fit in well with the job described, new characteristics that you may bring into the group, and also be aware of areas where you may need additional training and experience so you can present them in a positive proactive way when they come up in the discussion.*
What is the primary interest of the employer? What is the structure of the group?	*You must learn about the group's structure and research interests and be aware of their published work. Check the web page of the company or university, their newsletters and brochures, their annual activity reports, or as we said above, google them.*
What are the main strengths of the group? What are the main needs of the group?	*From your research into the group, you must be able to highlight a list of the main strengths of the group, which are part of your reasons for applying, and which you will be asked about at the interview. Also, you may want to identify areas of concern for you as an employee. If you have applied for the post we should safely assume that there were not many of these. Identifying needs, in addition, gives you the chance to create niches for you to fill in with your experience.*
Who will *be* forming the interview panel? How formal (or informal) is the *atmosphere* of the interview likely to be?	*You must learn about any additional members of the interview panel (e.g., colleague members of the group, human resources, university staff...) and get a sense of how formal or informal the interview will be.*

Questions you will be asked at the interview

Tell us about yourself	*This is a classic, and you must have an articulate answer well rehearsed and ready. Do not simply repeat your résumé point by point; they have that information already and it is not what they are looking for. Do not provide them either with every little personal detail of your life that may bear no relevance for the purpose of the interview. Go something in between: what they want is a blend, a dialogue between your main work accomplishments and some relevant specific details of your personal life in relation to how the work accomplishments came about, and your general plans for the future. They want to put a personal face to the information on your résumé, and want to get to know the person behind the job. Deep down, what they want to know is whether they like you (professionally and personally). So, this is your chance to show them.*
What are your main strengths? What was your main accomplishment in your previous job?	*You must prepare answers for these questions. Obviously, under no circumstances you should brag or show off, no matter how strong your background is to support it. But on the other hand, you have to talk in a positive and professional way about your assets and strengths, and you have to show them that you stand firm by your accomplishments. The employers need that additional information that they couldn't get from your résumé to help them make a fully informed decision about the right candidate for the post. Remember that presenting yourself in a job interview in a negative way that apologizes for the things you haven't done rather than making a strong case for the things you have done is not a sign of honesty. It is sign of plain stupidity.*
What are your weaknesses? What do you consider to be the main gap in your training and experience?	*You are likely to be asked this as well. So, you better prepare an answer in advance. You may want to identify in your background areas for improvement that will be strengthened by the new job, but which are not main assets required to carry it out successfully. Show commitment to your own improvement that does not put in danger being competitive for the post.*
Why did you leave your last job?	*Just one piece of advice here: It would be a terrible mistake to use the answer to this question as an opportunity to condemn your past employer. Mention difficulties in passing, in a general and detached way, and put the stress on positive actions such as career progression and new challenges.*

(continued)

Do you prefer working alone or with others?	*The right answer is always the latter. Think of examples you can provide from your work history (e.g., students trained, joint ventures with colleagues, combined projects...). Do not completely rule out, however, mentioning your level of independence and autonomy, as a positive asset, but within the structure of the group.*
Why do you want to work with us? What about our lab most appeals to you? What is it that you expect from this job?	*This is not only your chance to flatter the* employer *(which it partly is), but also to show how their strengths as a group and the characteristics of the post are meaningful to you as part of your career progression*
What are your longer-term career objectives? How do you see yourself professionally in five years?	*One of these is just the natural next question that you will face after the one above. Be* modest *here (winning the Nobel Prize should not be an option), but clear about what kind of professional future and impact you see yourself having in the future.*

Questions you will have to be ready to ask the interviewers

What do you value the most and expect from an ideal candidate?

You already know some of that from the job description. Remember in our example: "Highly motivated, mature and responsible scientist committed to working in a competitive academic environment sought." Asking directly will give you a more natural and direct answer from the employer. The answer will give you guidance on how to present yourself to meet the ideal expectations as close as possible. You may want to try this question earlier in the interview if there is a chance.

Do you have any concerns about my capacity to perform the job and fit in? Is there anything else that you need from me to have a complete idea of my suitability for the post?

Hopefully they won't have any concerns. But if they do and you don't ask, those concerns will remain in their heads whether they are correct or not. Only if you bring them out in the open you will have an opportunity to solve them.

I have really enjoyed our discussion and am very interested in the opportunity to join your team. Is there anything else that you need from me to make a hiring decision?

I think I would be really good at the job. Do you think we could work it out?

These are examples of questions to the interview panel that allow you to gently express an interest in the position. In addition, these formulations call for some form of feedback from the interviewers in a smooth and positive way.

Is there any additional information about the job that you believe I should know before making a decision and that we haven't had a chance to discuss yet?

Defensive questions are sometimes necessary, and this is a fairly put question that brings you and the interviewer closer ("that you believe...", "that we haven't had a chance..."). It is reasonable to think that a mature candidate would want to rule out other reasons for concern that have not come up in the discussion. You could soften it a bit by adding an introduction statement of interest as in the questions above: "I have enjoyed our discussion and am very interested in the opportunity to join your team. Is there any additional information...").

Money, pension, health plan, and other benefits...

Without a doubt these are all critical aspects of any job negotiation. But you cannot negotiate with what you haven't obtained yet. Although these issues need to be discussed, we believe that you shouldn't initiate this discussion, and you will be in a stronger position to discuss them once they have shown interest in you and you have some form of a job offer.

UNIT XI

Unit XI   The Laboratory Environment

In this unit we take a look at the research laboratory environment in English. Our goal is to help you identify and refer correctly to various types of rooms, pieces of equipment, and other devices typically found in a biomedical research lab. Lack of fluency in this area may often be a source of frustration for non-native researchers, who need to point embarrassingly at or undertake convoluted descriptions of facilities that they cannot find the right word for. In addition, native English-speaking researchers face the baffling challenge of deciphering what their non-native English-speaking colleagues are trying to say.

This unit will increase your command of English terminology and scientific slang related to the lab, and will provide you with the tools to say and write exactly what you mean. It will boost your confidence and help you communicate with your colleagues more effectively when technical issues or difficulties arise and need to be sorted out.

Commonly Misused or Misunderstood Terms

There are technical terms used in laboratories that non-native English speakers often get wrong. Some words can be confusing even for native English speakers. For instance, the differences between a rocker and a shaker, or between a stir rod and a stir bar, might be elusive not only to foreign scientists but also to less experienced native ones. This first section of the unit attempts to demystify some common terms used in a biomedical laboratory setting that we have all too often stumbled over.

- *Instruments/Equipment*
  All instruments are equipment, but not all equipment comprises instruments. An instrument is a device used to record, measure, or process data. Equipment is apparatus needed to perform a task.
  For example, a thermometer is used to measure the temperature of a solution; therefore, it is considered an instrument. However, a hotplate is used to heat solutions. A hotplate does not measure or record data; therefore, it is not an instrument.

R. Ribes et al., *English for Biomedical Scientists*,
DOI: 10.1007/978-3-540-77127-2_11, © Springer-Verlag Berlin Heidelberg 2009

- *Rocker/Shaker*
  Both items are used to mix or agitate samples within flasks or tubes. However, a shaker moves in a rotating motion, whereas a rocker moves in a back-and-forth or side-to-side motion (like a cradle). A shaker is generally used to grow bacteria or yeast. A rocker is often used to mix contents in a test tube.

- *Weight/Mass*
  In everyday use, the terms weight and mass are often used interchangeably; however, this is incorrect. The difference between these two words can be quite confusing to many people. Weight can be defined as the force of gravity on an object. It is the force with which the earth pulls on the object. Mass, on the other hand, is the amount of matter in an object.

- *Balance/Scale*
  In everyday English, a 'balance' is often used as a synonym for a 'scale.' However, in technical or scientific context, the meaning of 'balance' and 'scale' are different. A balance is an instrument used to measure the weight of an object, whereas a scale is used to measure the mass of an object. The difference between weight and mass has been given above.

- *Lab book/Log book*
  Lab book (also known as a laboratory notebook) and log book have the same meaning: both are books to record day-to-day activities. In some laboratories, the terms 'lab book' and 'log book' are used interchangeably. However, in other laboratories a lab book and a log book have slightly different meanings: a laboratory book is a primary record of personal research and a log book is used to record the performance of equipment and track users of equipment. This type of log book is important for properly maintaining equipment.

- *Film wrap/Foil wrap*
  Film wrap (also known as cling film or plastic wrap) is a clear, thin, flexible plastic covering used to wind or fold around something. Foil wrap (also known as tin foil) is thin aluminium covering used to wrap around something. For example, aluminium foil can be used to cover flasks prior to autoclaving. Film wrap can be used to wrap membrane filters or other blots to keep them from drying out.

- *Spray bottle/Wash bottle*
  A spray bottle has a trigger pump and nozzle; however, it is not a pressurized container. For example, most window and glass cleaners come in spray bottles. Unlike the spray bottle, a wash bottle is a squeeze dispensing bottle with an angled spout; one must squeeze the bottle to draw out fluid. This type of bottle is often used to rinse beakers or lab benches.

- *Oven/Incubator*
  It can be difficult to distinguish visually between an oven and incubator since they often look very similar. The difference between the two is the maximum temperature specification. Incubators generally have maximum temperatures

of up to 100°C, whereas lab ovens usually have a maximum temperature of around 200–300°C. Laboratory ovens are often used for drying glassware or purging glassware of RNase activity. Incubators are often used for the culture of micro-organisms and animal cells.

- **Stir rod/Stir bar**
  Both are used to stir liquid in flasks or beakers. However, a stirring rod is a long slender cylinder made of glass or chemical resistant plastic used to stir solutions by hand. A stir bar is a small, white, plastic-coated magnet often used in conjunction with a plate stirrer.

- **Scalpel/Blade/Razor**
  A scalpel is a small, straight, thin-bladed knife used in dissections. It consists of a blade and a handle. A blade is the cutting part of a knife, whereas a razor is a cutting instrument used to shave unwanted hair from the skin.

- **Scoopula/Spatula**
  A scoopula is a rolled-up stainless-steel utensil with one bevelled end and one blunt end. It is generally used to transfer a small quantity of solid compounds from a container into a weighing vessel. A spatula is a flat, thin utensil used for spreading, mixing, or scooping substances.

- **Light box/UV transilluminator**
  Both are box-shaped devices that contain lamps mounted within the box and have a white-glass or plastic cover. Both devices provide an illuminated viewing surface for fine detailed inspections. However, a light box uses white light to view items, such as autoradiography films, transparencies, cultures, etc. In contrast, a UV transilluminator uses UV light to view DNA/RNA in agarose gels stained with ethidium bromide.

- **Hot plate/Heat block**
  A hot plate is a small device used to heat solutions in glass beakers, flasks, bottles, and other glassware. It has a flat work surface so that it can be used with a variety of sizes of glassware. Unlike a hot plate, a heat block is a device that does not have a flat surface; instead it has holes where tubes can be inserted. It is used to heat samples in tubes. Most heat blocks can accommodate various tube sizes.

Here are a few technical terms used in most laboratory settings that have virtually the same meaning and that you may find are often used interchangeably:

- **Coverslip/Cover glass/Cover slide**
  All are protectors that are placed over specimens on microscope slides. They come in three basic shapes: circular, square, or rectangular.

- **Weighing dish/Weigh boat**
  Both are used for handling solid or liquid samples, especially for general purpose weighing. They come in various shapes. Weighing dishes are often referred to as ones that are circular in shape.

- *pH Paper/pH Strip*
  Both terms describe special paper used to measure the acidity or alkalinity of a solution. The only difference between these terms is that a pH strip describes a narrow piece of pH paper.

- *Table-top/Bench-top*
  Both words are normally used as adjectives to describe equipment that can be used on top of a table or bench. These two words are used to describe equipment made or designed to operate while sitting on a table or work bench. For example, bench-top or table-top centrifuges are smaller and compact compared to floor-model centrifuges.

- *Fume hood/Fume cupboard/Chemical hood*
  All describe the same thing: a partially enclosed workspace or piece of equipment designed to keep hazardous gases and vapors away from the work atmosphere and limit personnel exposure to hazardous fumes.

Types of Biomedical Research Laboratories

Laboratories are generally classified as wet, dry, or combined wet/dry:

- Wet laboratories or spaces are areas fitted with appropriate plumbing and ventilation, such as sinks, tap water, purified water, gas/vacuum lines, chemical storage, etc. Hands-on experimentation generally occurs in such laboratories.
- Dry laboratories or spaces are areas that do not have sinks or drains. These types of laboratories involve work with computers and state-of-the-art instruments, such as confocal and electron microscopes. Multidisciplinary fields such as bioinformatics and computational biology tend to use dry laboratories.
- Biomedical research facilities generally house combined wet/dry laboratories. Research carried out in biomedical research laboratories require specialized observation space used to house powerful computers and sophisticated software to process and analyze data generated by wet-lab experiments. For example, a researcher will prepare his sample in a wet space and analyze his sample using a confocal microscope in an adjacent room (a dry space).

Rooms Within a Large Laboratory

Laboratory space is generally partitioned into a large main room and several smaller rooms. Most experimental work is carried out in the main room; however, specific activities or experiments must be carried out in a separate room. Below is a list of rooms found in a typical research laboratory.

- *Controlled-environment rooms* are rooms with special temperature and humidity control. These include cold rooms and warm rooms.
  - A *cold room* is a walk-in refrigerator that generally operates at a temperature of 4°C.

○ A *warm room* is a room that generally operates at a temperature of 37°C and at a constant humidity. Warm rooms are often used to grow bacterial cultures.

- *Darkrooms* are light-tight rooms where light cannot penetrate when the door is closed. Dark rooms are generally used for light-sensitive activities, such as developing film. This type of room is usually equipped with a small red safelight so one can see in the dark while carrying out light-sensitive experiments. A "darkroom in use" sign is provided outside this room. This sign is hard-wired to the safelight, so when the safelight is turned on, the "darkroom in use" sign is illuminated. This lets other researchers know that someone is working on a light-sensitive activity or experiment in the darkroom (i.e., do not dare to attempt opening the door).

- *Radioactive rooms* are enclosed areas where radioactive work is performed. These rooms are often secured, access is strictly controlled, and the doors are normally locked. Access is restricted at all times from anyone not authorized to use radioactive isotopes. Only personnel that have undergone radiation training can have access to this type of room. A radioactive room can also be referred to as a 'hot room.' Hot room is an informal term for radioactive room.

- *Tissue culture rooms* are equipped to perform in vitro culture of cells or tissue cultures, which normally includes one or more tissue culture hoods, an incubator, a water bath, a bench-top centrifuge, and an inverted phase microscope.

- *Microscope rooms* house one or more microscopes to evaluate tissues and/or cultures at the cellular level.

- *Storage rooms* are small enclosed spaces where unused equipment or excess consumables are stored or kept until needed. It is similar to a closet in a house, only bigger.

Laboratory Equipment and Consumables

Glassware Commonly Found in a Laboratory

Each piece of laboratory glassware has a name and a purpose. Being a scientist, you probably already know the purpose of each piece of glassware pictured below. However, you may not know the correct English names for them. Use the images below to learn the English names of different types of laboratory glassware. Please note that some of the glassware listed below can be made of plastic for cost and convenience reasons.

The most common laboratory glassware items are pictured in the figure below:

Commonly Used Laboratory Consumables

Consumables in a lab refer to items that must be replaced regularly because they are used up. Most consumables in a lab are disposable items, meaning that they are designed to be thrown away after each use (or after several uses). Below is a

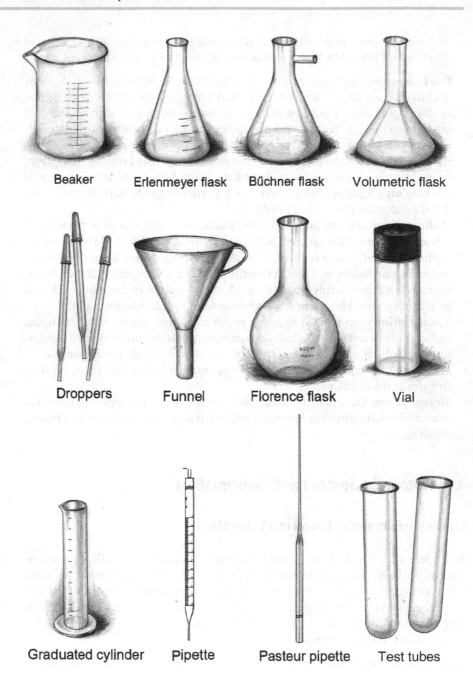

Beaker   Erlenmeyer flask   Büchner flask   Volumetric flask

Droppers   Funnel   Florence flask   Vial

Graduated cylinder   Pipette   Pasteur pipette   Test tubes

list of common consumables that you will need to find for daily experiments, ask the lab technician to order for you, or refer to in order to describe procedures and read or write research protocols.

- **Cell scraper** is a device with a rigid plastic blade on a handle. It is used to remove cells from a rigid substrate, such as a tissue culture dish or flask.
- **Cell culture dishes or tissue culture plates** are used to culture cells (normally adherent cells) in vitro. These dishes are generally circular in shape and have lids to protect contaminants from entering them. These dishes are completely transparent (clear) so you can look at your cells under a microscope.
- **Cell culture flasks** are also used to culture cells (normally in suspension) in vitro. The body of these flasks generally has a rectangular shape. They also have a small neck opening with a removal cap, which occasionally has a vent (vented flasks) for gas exchange.
- **Cuvettes** are small, transparent, square tubes and can come with or without lids depending on the type of cuvette:
  - **Electroporation cuvettes** are the type of cuvettes used in molecular biology as a way of introducing foreign substances, such as DNA, RNA, etc., into a cell. This type of cuvette has a removable lid.
  - **Spectroscopic cuvettes** are used to hold samples for spectroscopic reading of DNA, RNA, and proteins. This type of cuvette often does not have a lid.

- **Filter** is a porous paper used to remove particles and bacteria from a liquid sample. In biomedical research, filters are often used to sterilize solutions, such as media and buffers that contain heat-sensitive proteins since autoclaving may denature them. Solutions containing antibiotics, growth factors, or certain chemicals (such as SDS) are often filter sterilized. The following are examples of different types of filter supplies:
  - **Bottle-top filters** are filters that are mounted securely onto glass or plastic bottles.
  - **Syringe filters** are filters that are screwed securely onto syringes. These are designed to filter small amounts of liquid samples.

- **Inoculation loop** (also called **smear loop** or **wand**) is a circular-shaped wire (loop) with a handle. It is used to isolate pure bacteria colonies. Inoculation loops are generally made of metal; however, you can also find individually wrapped, single-use, plastic ones.
- **Microplate** is a plate of standardized size with a large number of wells, typically 96 or 384, arranged in orderly rows. The large number of wells allows for many different reactions to be carried out at the same time. These plates are often used for immunoassays, ELISA, etc.
- **Petri dishes** are generally used to culture bacteria. These dishes look very similar to tissue culture dishes. Petri dishes can also be used to culture animal cells as long as you coat these dishes with an extracellular matrix, such as collagen, laminin, or lysine, to allow anchorage-dependent cells to attach to the plates.

- *Slides*
  - *Microscope slides* are flat pieces of glass or plastic used to place specimens on to observe under a microscope.
  - *Cover slides* are used to cover specimens on a microscope slide.
- *Tubes* are cylindrical structures that hold liquid samples. Tubes come in a variety of sizes and for a wide variety of uses.
  - *Centrifuge tubes* are designed for use in floor centrifuges.
  - *Microcentrifuge tubes* are designed for use in bench-top centrifuges.
  - *Cryogenic tubes* are designed for the storage of biological material (such as cell lines and tissues) at cryogenic temperatures (approximately −190°C).
  - *PCR tubes* are specifically designed for use in PCR machines. These tubes are generally certified as RNase, DNase, and pyrogen free.

Commonly Used Laboratory Instruments

As mentioned above, lab instruments are devices used to record, measure, or process data. Here, we give you an overview in English of the most common types of instruments you may need to be familiar with.

- A *sequencer* is an instrument used to determine the sequence, usually DNA or protein, of a biological sample. DNA sequencer is used to determine the exact order of bases in a DNA molecule. A protein sequencer is used to determine the exact order of amino acids in a protein.
- A *thermometer* measures temperature. It is a glass tube sealed at both ends containing mercury or alcohol that expands or contracts as the temperature rises or falls. Most laboratories no longer use mercury thermometers because mercury poses a serious health risk and can harm the environment if released.
- *Scales* and *balances* are instruments used for weighing objects.
- A *timer* is an instrument used for measuring and signaling the end of a given interval of time.
- A *pH meter* is an instrument used to measure the pH (acidity or alkalinity) of a liquid.
- A *Pipetter* (also called pipette) is an instrument used to measure and transfer small, precise volumes of liquid.
- A *Spectrophotometer* is an instrument used to measure how much light of a given wavelength is absorbed by a liquid sample. This instrument is often used to estimate sample purity and concentrations of DNA, RNA, and protein samples.
- *Cell Counter* (also known as a Hemocytometer) is the simplest and cheapest device used to count cells in a sample. It is a modified microscope slide that has a counting chamber engraved in it. The volume of the chamber is known. A dye (such as Trypan blue) can be added to distinguish between live and dead cells.

- **FACS** (Fluorescence Activated Cell Sorter) is an instrument used to separate fluorescent labeled cells in a suspension based on size and fluorescence.
- **Microscopes** are instruments used for viewing objects so small in size that they are undetectable to the naked eye. The commonest types of microscopes used in biomedical research are the compound microscope, electron microscope, confocal microscope, and dissecting microscope. The cartoon below will provide you with the correct names for the main parts of a standard compound microscope.

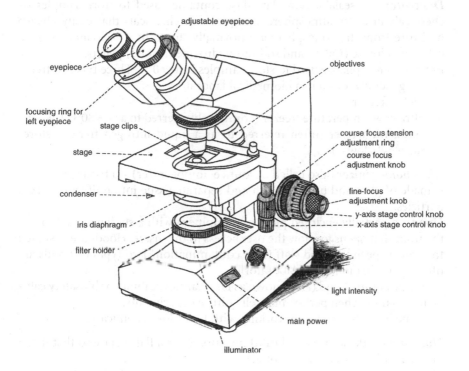

Commonly Used Laboratory Equipment

One of the challenges non-native English speakers must face when working in an English-speaking laboratory is learning the names of all the lab equipment. It would be nearly impossible to list all the possible lab equipment found in biomedical laboratories. The list below attempts to include the commonest items.

- **Autoclave** – a machine designed to sterilize solutions, glassware, and other laboratory objects by pressurized steam.
- **Laboratory water bath** – often referred to simply as "water bath," is a tank that keeps water at a precise and constant temperature. It is generally used to incubate bottles of culture media, samples in tubes, etc. Several water baths, each set at a different temperature, are often found in biomedical laborato-

ries. For example, restriction enzyme digestion of genomic DNA using EcoRI is often carried out in a 37°C water bath (or simple "37°C bath").

- **Bunsen burner** – a small, widely-used piece of equipment that produces a single smokeless gas flame. The size of the flame can be easily adjusted by the user. It is often used in microbiology laboratories to create a small, sterile work area since the heat from the flame creates a draft moving upwards, thus preventing contents from falling into the area.
- **Cryostat** – a microtome kept at very low temperatures. It is used to cut very thin sections of a frozen specimen for microscopic examination.
- **Desiccator** – a sealable, circular, glass container used to store samples or chemicals in a dry atmosphere. Samples and chemicals that easily absorb moisture from the atmosphere are normally stored in a desiccator, such as calcium chloride ($CaCl_2$) and sodium hydroxide (NaOH) pellets.
- **Freezer** – an appliance used to store samples below 0°C. Three types of freezers are generally found in a biomedical laboratory:
  - −20°C freezer
  - Ultra-low temperature freezer (commonly referred to as a −80°C freezer)
  - Cryogenic freezer (often referred to as a liquid nitrogen freezer) stores samples below −150°C

- **Glass homogenizer** (also called a Dounce homogenizer) – a tissue grinder. It is made of glass and used to crush and separate tissue into uniformed-sized particles.
- **Hood** – a partially enclosed piece of equipment with a sliding glass door on the front that opens to allow the user access to the inside. Hoods are designed to protect specimens and staff from contamination. Two types of hoods are often found in biomedical laboratories:
  - Tissue culture hood (also known as laminar flow cabinet or biosafety cabinet) is used when performing cell culture experiments.
  - Fume hood is used when working with hazardous chemicals.

- **Hot plate** – a device used to heat things up. It has a flat surface so that it can be used with a variety of sizes of glassware.
- **Centrifuges** – come as either "floor-model" centrifuges, which are larger centrifuges mounted on the floor, or as "bench-top" centrifuges, which are small, compacted centrifuges that can be operated on the bench or table.
- **Incubator** – a heated enclosed apparatus providing a controlled environment. Temperature, humidity, oxygen, and carbon dioxide can be controlled. At least three types of incubators are normally found in a biomedical laboratory:
  - Microbiology incubators are used to grow bacterial cultures.
  - Tissue culture incubators (also known as CO_2 incubators) are designed to provide optimal growth conditions for cells and tissues.
  - Hybridization incubators (also known as hybridization ovens) are used to incubate experiments which require two complementary strands of nucleic acids to bind or anneal. Examples of such experiments include Northern Blotting, Southern blotting, library screening, colony or plaque screening, and in situ hybridization.

- *Microtome* – a device used to cut a biological specimen into thin slices, at room temperature, for microscopic examination.
- *Refrigerator* (or *fridge*) – an appliance used to store samples normally at approximately 4°C.
- *Rotary evaporator* (can be informally referred to as a *Rotavap*) – a device used to quickly remove water from a mixture. A rotary evaporator generally found in biomedical laboratories looks very similar to a bench-top centrifuge. It spins and heats your sample under a vacuum.
- *Sonicator* – a device using high-frequency sound waves, to separate tissue into uniformed-sized particles or to dissolve samples completely.
- *Thermal Cycler* (or *PCR machine*) – an instrument used to amplify specific regions of DNA by the polymerase chain reaction.
- *UV-light box* (also known as a *transilluminator*) – used to visualize DNA bands in an agarose gel stained with Ethidium bromide (EtBr).
- *UV crosslinker* – a device used to expose samples to specific amounts of UV radiation. It is often used to fix DNA or RNA to membranes or blots.
- *Vibrocutter* – a device used to cut a biological specimen into thin slices, by an oscillating blade, for microscopic examination.
- *Vortex mixer* – an instrument used to mix small vials of liquid. The surface of the vortex mixer moves rapidly in a circular motion.

Unit XII   Laboratory Writing

Several units in this book thus far have been devoted to scientific writing. From the writing of scientific manuscripts (Unit IV) and specific scientific correspondence (Unit V) to curriculum vitae and cover letters (Unit IX). As important as the writing of manuscripts, letters, or CVs is, as a whole it only represents a small proportion of the actual writing that any scientist does. Your major initial writing challenge as a non-native scientist working in an English-speaking lab is everyday laboratory writing. You will have to be able to keep accurate and clear records of your work, make entries in laboratory notebooks, write concise clear lab protocols, describe the preparation of reagents and solutions, or even more simply, prepare a lab report or write short informative notes. We thought it would be useful to devote a section of this book to these writing tasks. Such is the focus on this unit.

Scientific Protocols

A written record of a standard procedure used in a laboratory is known as a scientific protocol. It's a step-by-step instruction of how a particular technique in the lab is performed. Well-written protocols are also used to ensure researchers within a lab carry out standard procedures correctly and in the same way in order to reduce sources of variation within their experimental results. It improves lab work consistency.

Here are some general guidelines for writing scientific protocols:

- Write protocols in a concise, step-by-step chronological order, and easy-to-follow format. They should be easy for the reader to understand and follow.
- Use short, plain, and direct sentences or bullets, since the person reading the protocol must read and carry out the experiment simultaneously.
- Use the imperative (command) or present tense. Protocols are explicit technical instructions that the reader must do.
- Begin sentences with an active verb.

R. Ribes et al., *English for Biomedical Scientists*,
DOI: 10.1007/978-3-540-77127-2_12, © Springer-Verlag Berlin Heidelberg 2009

For example,

  "*Add* two grams of NaCl to a 50-ml flask."

  NOT

  "Two grams of NaCl is added to a 50-ml flask"

Other examples:

  "*Transfer* supernatant to new tubes…"
  "*Inoculate* 50 ml of LB with…"
  "*Centrifuge* for 5 min in a microcentrifuge at 1000× (g) to remove…"
  "*Precipitate* the DNA at room temperature by adding…"

The table below is a list of commonly used active verbs in scientific protocols.

Add	Construct	Make	Rinse
Adjust	Discard	Measure	Standardize
Agitate	Dissect	Mix	Stimulate
Analyze	Dissolve	Obtain	Store
Aspirate	Estimate	Place	Take
Assemble	Fill	Pulverize	Turn off
Balance	Filter	Quantify	Use
Calculate	Label	Record	Wash
Collect	Locate	Remove	Weigh

- Use visual aids such as graphs, pictures, diagrams, and flow charts when possible. In technical scientific writing, a picture is indeed worth many more than a thousand words.
- Include all essential steps with sufficient detail so that the reader is able to follow the instructions and perform the protocol successfully and consistently. However, avoid excess unnecessary detail.

Here is an example of a commonly used protocol:

Tail DNA Extraction

1. Place a small tail sample into a 1.5-ml microcentrifuge tube.
2. Add 0.5 ml Tail Extraction buffer containing 0.5 mg/ml Proteinase K.
3. Incubate at 56°C overnight.
4. Add 200 µl 6M ammonium acetate to the sample and vortex briefly.
5. Incubate sample on ice for 10–15 min.
6. Centrifuge at full speed for 10 min in a microcentrifuge.
7. Transfer supernatant to a clean microcentrifuge tube containing 500 µl 100% isopropanol and mix thoroughly by repeated inversions.

8. Centrifuges ample for 3 min.
9. Wash DNA with 70% ethanol and centrifuge for 3 min.
10. Remove 70% ethanol and allow DNA to dry partially.
11. Add 100 μl TE buffer.

Lab Notebook Entries

A lab notebook is the primary record of a researcher's work. All data, detailed observations, and results from each experiment are written in this type of book. The purpose of a laboratory notebook is to keep track of what you have done and the results you have obtained, and to communicate it effectively enough so that a second party can read and understand the analysis and, if necessary, repeat the experiment exactly or be able to continue and extend the work. Thus, neatness, accuracy, clarity, and directness should always be your main focus when writing in laboratory notebooks.

There are a lot of ways and rules for keeping a laboratory notebook. You should always apply the rules of the organization where the experiments are conducted. If the organization where you work has no specific rules and regulations regarding notebook entries then use the guidelines suggested in this section.

General Guidelines for Notebook Keeping

- Each lab notebook should be used by only one single researcher.
- All pages in lab notebooks should be consecutively numbered, and
- Permanently bound to show that no pages were removed, thus avoiding the question of missing data. Most lab notebooks come with pre-numbered pages.
- Reserve the first few pages of the notebook for a Table of Contents. This is a list of experiments performed and the page numbers on which they start.
- Laboratory notebooks should always be written in permanent ink. Mistakes are not to be erased but should be crossed out with a single horizontal line. The error should still be readable.
- All entries should be recorded in chronological order. If you are carrying out two experiments at once then use continuation notes. Make a note on the last page of the unfinished experiment as to the page where it will continue. Make a note to previous pages too.
  For example,
  "Continue on page XX" is a reference to a subsequent page.
  "Continued from page X" is a reference to a previous page.
- All entries must be legible. Try to keep your notebook with the idea that someone else must be able to read and understand what you have done. The notebook should always be up-to-date because it can be collected at any time

by the institution you work for. In English-speaking countries, laboratory notebooks are generally, if not always, owned by the institution or company where the work is carried out.

- All entries should be accurate and detailed. Include successful and unsuccessful experiments. Write down the names of people who provided assistance. However, do not make entries that are not related to your project.
  For example,
     "Confirm squash with Bronwen, Wed 21st at 18:00."

- Loose raw data (such as spreadsheets, print-outs, photographs) can be either affixed to the pages of your notebook or kept in a separate folder or binder. If loose data is not affixed to your notebook then it is necessary to cross referencet hem.

- Introduce each experiment with a title and purpose. The purpose is the reason or goal of the experiment. It should only be one or two sentences long.
  For example,
  Title: "Confirmation and characterization of BAC clones."
     Purpose: "To ensure that the BAC clone stocks sent by UK HGMP Resource Centre were pure and contained the desired gene, and to determine the size of the upstream and downstream regions from the desired gene in each BAC clone."

- Protocols should be written in full. When the same protocol is carried out more than once, then there is no need to write it again. Just refer to the location of the full description and only note the changes you make to the protocol.
  For example,
  "Tail DNA Extraction protocol was used (see page 24). Tail DNA was resuspended in 50 µl TE (instead of 100 µl)."

- Data should be written in past tense. In general, personal pronouns should be avoided.
  For example,
     "Embryos containing the Sox10-GFP transgene exhibited green fluorescence in the CNS."
  NOT
     "I saw green fluorescence in the CNS of embryos containing the Sox10-GFP transgene."

- Include your interpretation/comments/ideas about the data or procedure. This is generally very brief.
- All entries must be dated. When writing in lab notebooks, a common mistake which leads to confusion is the writing of calendar dates in all-numeric form, since this format varies in different parts of the world. In the UK, the date is read as DAY/MONTH/YEAR, whereas in the US it is read as MONTH/DAY/YEAR.
  For example,
  02/08/08
  In the UK, this would read as the 2nd of August 2008

In the US, this would read as the 8th of February 2008
It is always best to spell out the month, either in full or in the abbreviated form:
August 2, 2008 or Aug. 2, 2008
February 8, 2008 or Feb. 8, 2008

Below is a good example of a laboratory notebook entry:

Title of Experiment/Study *Genotyping Sox10-Cre transgenic mice*   Book No **3**   Page 163

Other references   Date **Oct. 24, 2007**

To determine which mice from litter 36 carry the Sox10-Cre transgene.

Tail biopsies were obtained from 3 week old mice.
Tail DNA Extraction protocol was used (see page 156).

PCR rxn mix	×15	PCR amplification condition
Taq 0.2 μl	3	(Program GAPI 62)
10× buffer 2.5 μl	37.5	
25 mM MgCl₂ 1.5 μl	22.5	94 °C 4 min 1 cycle
20 mM dNTP 0.25 μl	3.75	94 °C 30 sec
Primer 1 0.1 μl	1.5	56 °C 50 sec 35 cycles
Primer 2 0.1 μl	1.5	72 °C 2 min
H₂O 19.35 μl	290.25	72 °C 10 min 1 cycle
Tail DNA 1.0 μl	—	
total: 25 μl		

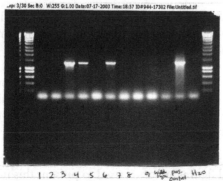

xp: 3/30 Sec B:0   Wi:255 G:1.00 Date:07-17-2003 Time:18:57 ID#944-17302 File:Untitled.tif

1 2 3 4 5 6 7 8 9 wild pos. H₂O
type control

PCR was successful. Pups 3, 4, and 6 carry the transgene.

Laboratory Reports

This section is designed particularly for students and researchers at very early stages in their scientific careers. In these early stages, laboratory reports are a common way to document your findings and communicate their significance. Different professors/tutors/lab heads have different rules about the style or format of a laboratory report. Here we provide you with a general guideline on how to write a laboratory report that will have to be adapted to the specific settings of your lab.

Lab reports are generally divided into the following sections:

- Title Page
- Aim/Objective
- Introduction
- Material & Methods
- Results
- Discussion
- Conclusion
- References

Title Page is the first page of the report. The title of the experiment, your full name, instructor or supervisor's name, and date should be included.

Aim is the purpose of the experiment.
Here are examples of expressions used in this section:
"The aim of this experiment/practical is to determine…"
"To investigate the effects of…"
"To determine if …"
"To measure…"
"To verify…"

Introduction is an overview of what the experiment is about. It is used to inform the reader about the topic of the report. It should contain relevant background information that may be needed to make sense of the information in the report.

Material & Methods is a description of the procedures used to collect data in the experiment. In reports, protocols should always be written in complete sentences and should be written in past tense.
For example,

"All sections were mounted on glass slides and air-dried for at least 1 hour, and either stored at −80°C or used immediately. After sections were air-dried, the slides were first immersed in 1× phosphate-buffered saline containing 0.1% Triton X-100 for 5 minutes to remove excess embedding medium."

Results section contains experimental data in a form that is easy to read and follow for the reader. Tables and figures are often used to present this information. All tables and figures should be numbered consecutively and should have a title and a brief description.

Below are examples of a table and a figure:

Table I. CCR7/CD45RA subset distribution of expanded antigen-specific CTL's.

CELL LINE	VIRUS Ag	EPITOPE	Tem CCR7– CD45RA–	Teff CCR7– CD45RA+	Tcm CCR7+ CD45RA–	Tn CCR7+ CD45RA+
1	CMV–pp65	NLV	89	1	5	5
2	CMV–pp65	NLV	69	26	2.5	2.5
3	CMV–pp65	NLV	70	27.5	1.25	1.25
4	CMV–pp65	NLV	52	35	10	3
5	EBV–EBNA3A	FLR	92	1.5	5	1.5
6	EBV–EBNA3A	FLR	76	3	7.5	14
7	EBV–EBNA3A	FLR	91	7	–	2
8	EBV–LMP2	CLG	59	1	24	16
9	EBV–LMP2	CLG	70	16	7	7
10	EBV–LMP2	CLG	46.5	17.5	13	23
11	EBV–LMP2	CLG	73	2	21	4
12	EBV–LMP2	CLG	34	14	9	43
13	EBV–LMP2	CLG	67	23	9	1
14	EBV–LMP2–	CLG	87	12	1	–

Tem: Effector memory; Teff: Terminal effectors; Tcm: Central memory; Tn: Naïve; Ag: Antigen

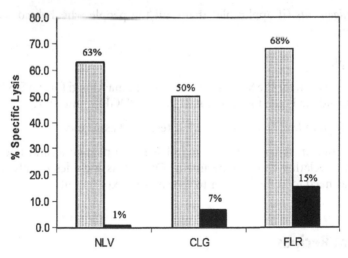

Fig. 1. Cytotoxic ^{51}Chrominum-release assay. Efficient lysis at E:T ratio of 10:1 mediated by CMV and EBV-specific CTL lines after 12 days culture with peptide-pulsed DC. CTL raised against HLA A2- restricted CMV epitope NLV and EBVLMP2a epitope CLG were incubated with NLV- and CLG-pulsed T2 cells respectively and peptide-pulsed PHA blasts were used as targets for HLA B8 restricted FLR-specific CTL. Hatched columns represent peptide-specific lysis and shaded columns non-specific lysis of unpulsed target cells.

Discussion section is where you interpret and discuss your results in detail. This section is generally long. Here you can discuss the validity of your results, how the experiment can be improved, the significance of the findings, and how they fit into current knowledge.

Conclusion states the outcome of the experiment in a few sentences. It should highlight the key findings in your report.

Reference section contains a list of all books and journals referred to in the text of your lab report. Although there are many ways to organize your references (see Unit IV), we would recommend keeping it simple in alphabetical order for a lab report.

Examples of cited papers:

MacKenzie, A., Abbott, J. and Macdonald, J.A. (2008) Identification and characterization of the mouse PDGFRα gene. Nature 800, 454-466.

Stronzo, S., Bennett, R.B., MacKenzie, A., Chang, L., Wang, F. and Miller, A. (2004) PAC modification and generation of Sox10-Cre transgenic mice. Genesis 64, 335-346.

An example of citing a reference in the body of your paper:

"EGFP expression was found to be expressed in a restricted region within the ventral telencephalon and spinal cord corresponding to known regions of OL specification (Stronzo et al., 2004)."

Acknowledgements (if applicable) thank all the people who helped with your experiment.

For example,

"I thank Dr. Sirolli for the Sox10-GFP embryos; Tina Alongi for the Sox10 in situ probe; and Adelia Frade for antibodies against PDGFRα and PLP."

"I am grateful to Marisa Di Prata for her technical assistance."

Appendix (optional) contains non-mandatory supplemental and background information relating to the experiment. Often this includes details that your reader may need to know in order to repeat your experiment

Reagent Recipes

A reagent recipe is a record of chemicals and the amounts needed to prepare a reagent or solution. Chemicals used are generally written in the order they are combined. *Stock conc.* refers to the concentration of the stock solution. A stock solution is a common reagent or chemical at a standardized concentration that needs to be diluted to a lower concentration for actual use. *Final conc.* refers to the working concentration of the chemical. Quantity needs to be specified as volume or weight. All reagent recipes must have a name to identify what you are making. The notes section is used to record information regarding storage conditions or any special care that must be taken into consideration. Scientists often write reagent recipes on blank cue cards.

Below you will find an example of a reagent recipe for TE buffer and Extraction buffer:

TE Buffer

Component	Stock Conc.	Final Conc.	Quantity
Tris (pH 7.5)	1 M	100 mM	50 ml
EDTA (pH 8.0)	0.5 M	1 mM	1 ml

Bring volume to 500 ml with ddH_2O
Notes: Autoclave solution and store at room temperature.

Tail EXTRACTION BUFFER

Component	Stock Conc.	Final Conc.	Quantity
Tris (pH 7.5)	1 M	100 mM	50 ml
EDTA (pH 8.0)	0.5 M	5 mM	5 ml
NaCl	5 M	200 mM	20 ml
SDS	10%	0.2%	10 ml

Make up volume to 500 ml with distilled H_2O
Notes: Autoclave solution before adding SDS. Store at room temperature.

Short Notes

When writing short informal notes or instructions, articles, subject or object pronouns, and prepositions are often left out. This is usually done in order to save time or space.

Sample:

I am having lunch in the cafeteria. I will be back at 1:30 p.m. (long version)
Gone to lunch. Back at 1:30. (condensed version)

The above sentence has been condensed in just a few words; however, the essential message/point is clear.

Unit XIII Laboratory Safety and Biohazards

All laboratories have potential hazards, and the importance of understanding lab safety cannot be emphasized strongly enough. Scientists are expected to understand and be aware of the health and safety issues associated with their profession. Regardless of the standards for laboratory safety in their country of origin and regardless of their position, all researchers require a good understanding of safety features in English before they can begin working in an English-speaking laboratory. All research institutions in English-speaking countries require all new staff to go through a safety orientation or training course before they can begin work. Your employer or institution has a legal requirement to provide you with safety training before you begin work. Generally, a safety officer, a person who acts as the institutional or departmental administrator for safety-related matters, gives the course, and a written safety test must be completed by all new employees following training before work can commence in the laboratory. It is your legal duty to cooperate with your employer or institution's efforts to improve safety in the workplace. Not respecting safety regulations and procedures while working in a laboratory does not only put your own health and others' at risk, but it may also have an impact on the lab's license and may lead to disciplinary action against you. Everyone must be aware and responsible so we can all enjoy our research while staying safe!

In this chapter we aim to familiarize you with English vocabulary and symbols associated with laboratory safety and to give you some general safety guidelines. It is intended to help you address safety issues with confidence even under difficult and stressful circumstances such as emergency situations. This strong background knowledge on lab safety in English will make you more confident when you have to embark on the new experience of starting work in an English-speaking lab. Specific training requirements will not be discussed however, since they generally vary from country to country, between regions and localities within countries, and between institutions within localities.

In order to make you familiar with various aspects of biosafety in English, we have divided this unit into five sections: Personal protective equipment, Lab safety equipment, Chemical safety, Biological safety, and Radiation safety. Once you have finished reading this unit you can test your safety knowledge by taking the safety quiz located at the end of this chapter. An answer key is also provided.

R. Ribes et al., *English for Biomedical Scientists*,
DOI: 10.1007/978-3-540-77127-2_13, © Springer-Verlag Berlin Heidelberg 2009

Personal Protective Equipment (PPE)

It is vital that lab workers wear the correct protective equipment for the experiment they intend to carry out in order to avoid injury. Personal protective equipment includes lab coats (also known as white coats), safety glasses and goggles, face shields, gloves, and masks. When used properly, PPE minimizes personal exposure to hazardous material. Failure to use personal protective equipment is generally seen as a violation of safety rules or procedures.

Lab coats are loose knee-length white coats with deep pockets. Throughout the world, lab coats have become mandatory in research and medical institutions. They must be worn correctly at all times within laboratory areas and always be removed immediately on leaving the laboratory area. A badly stained or torn coat is a hazard and should be replaced immediately. Lab coats are generally provided and cleaned regularly by the institution at no charge.

Protective eyewear, as the name implies, protects the eye area in order to prevent particles or dangerous materials from entering the eye. Protective eyewear must always be worn whenever there is a chance of eye injury. Anyone working in or passing through areas that pose eye hazards should wear eye protection. Eye injuries in the laboratory are very common and can result in serious eye damage or blindness. Most forms of eye protection are light in weight and made from highly impact-resistant material (such as polycarbonate). The main types of protective eyewear are safety glasses, safety goggles, and face shields.

Safety glasses look just like regular eyeglasses; however, the lenses are more durable and provide better protection against flying debris. Safety goggles are different from safety glasses in that they are tight-fitting and have side shields and also provide an extra level of protection beyond safety glasses; they provide full coverage to the eyes. When safety goggles are worn correctly, they will provide protection to the eye and skin immediately surrounding the eyes from dust and splashes of liquid coming from any direction (above, below, side, or face-on). A face shield is a hard, clear plastic sheet that that covers the eyes and face completely. It generally covers the forehead, extends below the chin, and wraps around the side of face. It is intended to cover the entire face from accidental splashes of harmful liquids and some even protect against excessive exposure to ultraviolet radiation (to avoid a sunburned face). Not all face shields protect against UV; be sure that the item is specified by the manufacturer as providing protection at the wave length(s) you intend to use. The type of eye protection needed depends on the circumstances. For example, when the entire face needs protection, a face shield is used. It is important that you wear eye protection any time you are exposed to a potentially hazardous situation. For maximum protection, select the appropriate protective eyewear designed for the specific experiment you carry out and make sure you wear the appropriate eye protection throughout the entire experiment.

Hand protection: careful attention must be given to protecting your hands when working with potentially dangerous chemical or biological materials. Safety gloves are coverings used to protect the hands, with a separate part for each finger and thumb. Safety gloves are worn in biomedical research laboratories and animal rooms to protect the wearer from contact with damaging material. Gloves are provided by the laboratory for all its researchers. There are hundreds of different types of safety gloves. However, only a few different types of safety gloves are generally used in most biomedical research laboratories. Cryogenic gloves, heat resistant gloves, and chemical resistant gloves are the most common types found in biomedical laboratories. Cryogenic gloves are designed to provide protection to the hands from the dangers encountered when handling extremely cold items or substances, like liquid nitrogen. Liquid nitrogen can cause severe frostbites and cold burns. Gloves intended for liquid nitrogen use are generally not made to allow the hands to be put into the liquid. They only provide protection from accidental spills or contact with the liquid. These gloves are also designed to work with dry ice. Heat resistant protective gloves are designed to protect hands from intense heat and prevent heat burns. Biomedical research laboratories involved in RNA studies: glassware is often oven-baked at 200°C for at least 4 h to ensure it is free from enzymes that can degrade RNA (i.e., RNases). In order to remove glassware from these very hot ovens, one must use heat resistant gloves to protect hands from heat burns. Disposable chemical gloves are the most commonly used gloves in biomedical research laboratories and animal care facilities. These gloves may be made from latex, rubber, nitrile, polyvinyl alcohol (PVA), or polyvinyl chloride (PVC), etc. The type of chemical glove one will use should depend on the chemical being used. For example, nitrile gloves provide protection against oil based chemicals, whereas PVC gloves provide protection against aqueous chemicals. It is important to bear in mind that for chemical protection the wearer should determine the appropriate glove material to provide the desired protection. Some chemicals will rapidly penetrate some glove materials; therefore, incorrect selection or use of protective gloves can lead to chemical burns. One type of glove will not work in all situations.

Face masks, as the name implies, is a cover or partial cover for the face used for protection. It provides protective covering for the mouth and nose. Face masks generally found in biomedical research laboratories are called dust masks. These masks are the white disposable kind with two elastic bands, one that goes above the ears and the other below the ears. Dust masks block large airborne particles. They are often used when weighing out powders and during animal work. There are many different kinds of dust masks; therefore, know the limitation of the protection and wear the proper mask suitable for the job.

Laboratory Safety Equipment

The importance of understanding the types and use of safety equipment is essential to the practice of safe science. All employees are required to know how to use the available safety equipment before any emergencies occur. The majority of laboratories in English-speaking countries have access to the following basic safety equipment:

- *Emergency eyewash stations* provide on-the-spot elimination of accidental chemical or biological splashes to the eyes. They are designed to flush the eyes and face only.
- *Safety showers* provide on-the-spot removal of massive chemical or biological splashes on clothing or body. Safety showers are designed to have water sprayed over the entire body. Safety showers, however, are not designed to flush the user's eyes because the high rate or pressure of the water flow could cause damage.
- *Fire blankets* are, as the name implies, fire-resistant sheets of fabric that one uses to wrap around a person whose cloths are on fire.
- *Fire extinguishers* are essential portable fire-fighting tools used to control or put out small fires; however, they are not designed for large or spreading fires. There are different types of fire extinguishers, each of which are designed to put out different types of fires. The types and labeling of fire extinguishers vary among countries. For example, North America generally uses a picture labeling system to indicate which types of fires they are to be used on, whereas the UK uses a color coding system on their extinguishers. Using the wrong type of extinguisher can be dangerous; in some cases, it can cause a fire to spread. Therefore, it is extremely important to familiarize yourself in your institution with the types and labeling of fire extinguishers For example, water expelling type-A fire extinguishers should not be used on fires involving electrical equipment.

For your personal safety and the safety of others, you should know where the nearest fire extinguishers, fire alarm pull boxes, and fire exits are located. Fire alarm pull boxes are bright red boxes with handles generally located on walls near fire exits or in stairwells. In addition, you should know your institution's policy on fire safety. It is also important for the non-native English-speaking scientist to know that there are some common words associated with fire safety that are different in American and British English. For instance, a 'fire check' in Britain is a 'fire safety inspection' in America. The organization that is responsible for preventing and extinguishing unwanted fires is called a 'fire brigade' in Britain and a 'fire department' in America. A man or woman whose job is to stop unwanted fires is called a 'fireman' in Britain and a 'firefighter' in America. The building that houses the fire trucks or fire engines is called a 'fire station' in Britain and a 'firehouse' in America.

- *First Aid Kits* (also known as First Aid Box) contain emergency supplies for the treatment of unexpected minor injuries such as small cuts. Most first aid kits are labeled with a white cross on a green background; however, some kits are labelled with a red cross on a white background. First aid kits should be readily available to laboratory staff at all times. First aid kits can contain different items depending on the type of work performed in a laboratory. The names of the main contents found in a first aid kit are below:

- Adhesive strip (as known as 'bandage' or 'band aid' in North America and 'plasters' in the UK), is a material that you can place directly over a small cut in the skin in order to protect the wound and keep it clean. Various sizes are generally included in the kit.
- Various types and sizes of gauze dressing (or simply called gauze) — a cloth for covering a wound. It is usually made from cotton.
- Safety pins.
- Bottle of antiseptic solution.
- Eye pads.
- Disposable gloves.
- First aid book.
- Names of first aiders (these are people who have received basic training on how to give simple medical emergency treatment to injured persons) and how to contact them.

Chemical Safety

There are many hazards associated with working with chemicals. People who work with chemicals are required to know the hazards of the substances in their working area, and learn how to use them safely. Information on most substances is found on chemical safety data sheets, which are normally provided by the companies that you purchase your chemicals from. Laboratories should have a collection of safety data sheets for all chemicals found in their laboratory. Each chemical safety data sheet contains information, in a clear and concise manner, regarding a specific chemical such as physical data, recommended PPE, stability and reactivity, emergency and first aid procedures, health effects, toxicity, handling and storage, ecological information, and disposal considerations. Chemical safety sheets contain more data and information about the hazardous substance than the label found on the container holding the hazardous substance.

Chemical safety data sheet is also known as:

- Safety data sheet
- International chemical safety card (ICSC)
- Chemical safety card
- Product safety data sheet
- Material safety data sheet (MSDS)

What type of information will you find on a chemical label in English?

Labels are legal documents found on all hazardous substances. A label is the manufacturer's way of giving the user information about the product, telling you what the dangers are, and providing details about the supplier. Labeling requirements may differ from country to country; however, in most English-speaking countries labeling of any container that holds a hazardous substance is regulated by a governing body. These labels include basic information such as product name, ingredients, supplier's name, storage measures, reference to a MSDS, hazard symbols, risk phrases, precautionary measures, and first aid measures. It is extremely important to read and understand the label for the safe use of the hazardous substance. If you require more detailed information about the chemical you are using, you should refer to the MSDS. Labels contain basic information due to lack of space and therefore should not replace the MSDS.

Hazard symbols are often found on chemical labels. These symbols provide the user with a guide for quick recognition of the hazards associated with a specific chemical. A chemical might be labeled with more than one hazard symbol. One must be able to recognize and understanding the meaning of hazard symbols for the safe use of hazardous substances. The table below contains the Workplace Hazardous Materials Information System (WHMIS) classification of chemicals and their hazard symbols. There are six classes, several of which have subdivisions. Each class has a specific symbol to indicate the nature of the hazardous material, and includes a brief explanation of the type of danger they refer to.

Many different additional hazard symbols exist; however, a comprehensive review of all the symbols is beyond the scope of this unit. Those of you who want more information on hazard symbols can look at the websites located at the end of this unit. We also strongly recommend you to check your workplace safety manual or ask your safety officer.

Class	Symbol	Hazard	Description of Hazard
A		Compressed Gas	Contents under pressure (e.g., nitrogen)
B		Flammable and Combustible Material	May catch on fire easily in the presence of a spark or open flame (e.g., propane)
C		Oxidizing Material	May increase the risk of a fire or explosion when in contact with other combustible material

Class	Symbol	Hazard	Description of Hazard
D		Toxic or Poisonous Material	Materials causing immediate and serious toxic effects
D		Poisonous and Infectious Material	Materials causing other toxic effects
D		Poisonous and Infectious Material	Biohazardous infectious material
E		Corrosive Material	May cause chemical burns(e.g., acids, bases, phenols)
F		Dangerously Reactive Material	Materials that are very unstable and may explode as a result of shock, friction, or increase in temperature (e.g., benzoyl peroxide)

Biological Safety

There are many hazards associated with working with biological materials. The purpose of this section is to familiarize you with English vocabulary and usage associated with biological safety. Biological safety training is mandatory for those working in laboratories with biological agents. Learning the vocabulary associated with this area will pave your way to more easily learning your institute's biological safety policy. The main topics covered in this section of the chapter are genetically modified organisms risk assessment, biocontainment levels, biological safety cabinets, and disposal of biological waste.

- **Genetically Modified Organism (GMO) risk assessment** looks at the risk of infection from a GMO to humans, animals, and the environment. A genetically modified organism is an organism whose genetic material has been altered by gene technology. All projects involving GMOs are required to undergo a risk assessment before the project can begin. This generally involves submission of a GMO risk assessment form to the local GMO Safety Committee and approval of the risk assessment.

- **Biocontainment levels** are control measures used to lessen or completely prevent the escape of biological hazardous agents. There are four types of biocontainment levels. These four levels are designated as Biosafety Level (BSL) 1, 2, 3, and 4, Biosafety level 1 being the lowest BSL and level 4 the highest. A typical laboratory is a BSL 1 facility. BSL-1 is appropriate for working with micro-organisms that are not known to consistently cause disease in healthy adults (e.g., *E.coli*). BSL-2 is appropriate for working with micro-organisms that are known to cause mild disease to humans (e.g., Salmonella). BSL-3 is appropriate for micro-organisms that may be transmitted by the respiratory route which can cause serious and potentially lethal infection (e.g., SARS coronavirus). BSL-4 is appropriate for working with micro-organisms that pose a high risk of life-threatening disease and can be transmitted via the airborne route (e.g., Ebola virus). BSL-4 laboratories are difficult to design, build, and operate; therefore, most countries have only a few of these types of laboratories (e.g., Canada has two BSL-4 type laboratories; Australia and the UK both have three).
- **Biological safety cabinets** (or simply **hoods**) are safety equipment used to contain biological agents and protect the operator and the environment. These cabinets come in three different classes: class 1, 2, and 3:
  ○ Class 1 cabinets protect the operator from the biological agent but not the agent from the environment.
  ○ Class 2 cabinets provide protection to both the operator and the biological agent.
  ○ Class 3 cabinets are totally enclosed to prevent the release of airborne particles. This type of cabinet is designed to be completely air-tight in order to completely contain the hazardous material.
- **Biological Waste** Any unwanted solid or liquid materials that are contaminated with biological agents are referred to as biological waste (note, neither garbage nor rubbish, as we refer to discarded material outside the lab). Safe disposal of biological waste is extremely important to the health and safety of our environment. Improper disposal of this type of waste may cause infection to spread outside the laboratory. Policies for correct disposal of this type of waste can vary, and once again it is important for you to familiarize yourself with the rules and procedures for the proper disposal of biological waste in your institution.

Radiation Safety

In order to work with radioactive materials, the laboratory that you plan to carry out your radioactive experiments in will need to have a radiation permit (a license giving official permission) and you will need to attend a basic radiation safety training seminar.

Here are some terms you will encounter, the meaning of which may not be immediately obvious to the non-native English speaking scientist:

- **Radioactive dosimeter badges** (sometimes referred to as **film badges**) are used to monitor radiation exposure over an extended period of time. These badges are worn when working with or in areas where radioactive materials are being used. It is usually in the shape of a small badge or pack which is clipped to a person's laboratory coat. It is used to determine whether the radiation level one is exposed to falls within established safety limits.

- **Geiger counter** (also known as a **Survey meter**) is an instrument used to detect radiation in an area or object and measure its intensity. A tiny drop of contamination of a radioactive isotope can be easily detected with this instrument.

- **Plexiglas shields** are clear plastic materials used as protective barriers against radiation generated by beta-producing radioactive isotopes. These shields are placed between the user and the radioactive source. The most common beta-producing isotope used in biomedical research is 32 phosphorus (^{32}P). Plexiglas shields are not appropriate shields for gamma or X-ray producing sources.

- **Decontamination versus Decommissioning** – The use of these words in radiation protection may cause some confusion for non-English speaking individuals. Decontamination refers to the clean-up of loose or fixed surface radioactivity, whereas decommissioning is used when a radioactive work space or area is no longer used for radioactive work. See the examples below:
  - *All radioactive spills must be* decontaminated *using a special cleaning detergent.*
  - *The radioactive room was* decommissioned *and has now been transformed into a seminar room.*

Safety Quiz

In most English-speaking research institutions, a written safety test must be completed before one can begin doing research. The sample quiz below is an example of what you will find in your new workplace. Safety quizzes generally consist of true and false, multiple-choice, and spot the hazard-type questions. Taking the quiz below will allow you to test your knowledge gained in this chapter. Answers are located at the end of the quiz (see answer key).

The following quiz is made up of two parts: the true and false part and the multiple choice part.

Part 1:   Simply answer TRUE or FALSE to the following statements:

1) A laboratory coat is the standard minimum PPE in most laboratories. T/F
2) A white coat can be worn in common areas such as seminar rooms, staff rooms, and cafeteria. T/F
3) Latex gloves provide protection against all toxic chemicals and solvents. T/F
4) Class A water-based fire extinguishers should be used to control fires involving electrical equipment. T/F
5) Gloves should be selected on the basis of the material being handled. T/F
6) A person can be fired for asking questions about how to do their job safely or reporting unsafe working conditions? T/F
7) A radiation safety training course is often not mandatory for personnel who wish to work with radioactive materials. T/F
8) Geiger counters are used to monitor radiation exposure over an extended period of time. T/F
9) Plexiglas shields are protective barriers against all types of radiation. T/F
10) The following graphic symbol shown below indicates an oxidizing hazard. T/F

Part 2:   Choose the correct answer for each question. One answer only.

1) What would immediately be used if your clothing caught fire or if a large chemical spill had occurred on your clothing?
   A. Fire extinguisher
   B. Safety shower
   C. Laboratory sinks
   D. Eye-wash fountain

2) What should be done if a chemical gets in the eye(s)?
   A. Use the safety shower
   B. Immediately put your safety goggles on
   C. Immediately begin rinsing the eye(s) in the eye wash station
   D. Nothing, unless the chemical causes discomfort

3) What does PPE mean?
   A. Personal Protective Equipment
   B. Proper Protective Procedures

C. ProperP ersonal Equipment
D. Proper Procedures for Equipment

4) Class A fire extinguishers are suitable for:
A. Fire involving electrical equipment
B. Fire involving flammable liquids, such as petrol, oil, and diesel
C. Fire involving ordinary combustibles, such as wood, paper, and fabric
D. Fire involving flammable metals, such as aluminium, magnesium, and sodium

5) If the following symbol is depicted on a label, the material found in the container is:

A. Corrosive
B. Dangerously reactive
C. Irritant
D. Poisonous

6) Which item should not be found in a typical first aid kit?
A. Plasters
B. Prescription drugs
C. Disposable gloves
D. Safety pins

7) What does the following symbol mean?

A. Flammable
B. Oxidizer
C. Explosive
D. Compressed Gas

8) Chemical safety data sheets should be consulted:
A. If a hazardous material is ingested
B. Before working with a chemical
C. For the requirement of specific PPE
D. All the above

9) What does GMO mean?
   A. Genetically Modified Organisms
   B. General Modification of Organisms
   C. Genetic Model Organisms
   D. None of the above

10) Which type of fire extinguisher should NOT be used on a fire involving electrical equipment such as computers?
   A. Foam
   B. Water
   C. Dry chemical/powder
   D. CO_2

Answer key:

Part 1   1) T, 2) F, 3) F, 4) F, 5) T, 6) F, 7) F, 8) F, 9) F, 10) T
Part 2   1) B, 2) C, 3) A, 4) C, 5) D, 6) B, 7) A, 8) D, 9) A, 10) B

For further information about safety please see the websites below.

http://bmbl.od.nih.gov/ BSL U.S. Department of Health and Human Services Centres for Disease Control and Prevention and National Institutes of Health

www.hc-sc.gc.ca/ewh-semt/occup-travail/whmis-simdut/index-eng.php Health Canada

www.osha.gov/ U.S. Department of Labor Occupational Safety & Health Administration

http://hsis.ascc.gov.au/Default.aspx Australia's Hazardous Substances Information System

Unit XIV   Laboratory Animal Work

The use of animals has become essential for nearly all areas in modern biomedical research. Major advances in this field would not have been possible without their use. Today, the number of animal models genetically engineered for biomedical research is increasing rapidly.

The breeding, supply, and use of animals in research are highly regulated in English-speaking countries. For example, the Home Office (one of the most important UK government departments) is responsible for regulating animal research in the UK, and the US Department of Agriculture (a Federal Executive Department) is responsible for regulating the use and care of animals for scientific purposes.

Misunderstandings that violate animal work policies may result in professional misconduct, penalties, and even loss of all privileges to conduct animal research for the entire laboratory. Therefore, we thought it was important to write a chapter dedicated to animal research. This chapter is not intended to provide you with detailed regulations and protocols for the care and use of laboratory animals since this will vary among different countries and institutions. It will, however, focus on providing you with expressions, terminology, and general guidelines commonly used among researchers, animal facility staff, and veterinarians.

What Is Animal Research?

The use of animals in scientific experiments is called animal research. It includes any scientific procedure, test, investigation, or study involving animals. Animal experimentation generally falls into one or both of the following two types: basic research and applied research. Basic animal research is carried out with a focus on the discovery of nature as it is, the way it works or evolves. The main goal is knowledge on its own. Applied research shifts the focus onto using our knowledge to solve practical problems. Consider the following questions:

R. Ribes et al., *English for Biomedical Scientists*,
DOI: 10.1007/978-3-540-77127-2_14, © Springer-Verlag Berlin Heidelberg 2009

Where do fat cells (adipocytes) arise from?
How does the mammalian brain develop during embryogenesis?
How does the hippocampus contribute to memory?
What is the most effective drug against HIV?
Can angiogenesis inhibitors destroy fat tissue?
Can caffeine protect against Alzheimer's?

The first three questions are examples of questions asked in basic research and the last three are examples of questions asked in applied research.

Animals commonly used in research are non-human primates, cats, guinea pigs, fish, frogs, rabbits, mice, and rats. Mice and rats make up 80%–90% of all animals used in biomedical research. They make good research subjects for a variety of reasons: they are genetically close to humans, they are small in size, they are relatively inexpensive to breed and maintain, and they reproduce large litters. In addition, mice and rats have short life cycles so they can be easily studied throughout their whole life span or across several generations.

Animal Work Licences

Scientists wishing to carry out research involving live animals must seek the necessary licences before starting any animal work. Carrying out research involving animals is considered unlawful without a licence in English-speaking countries. It is your responsibility to familiarize yourself with the laws in the particular country where you wish to carry out animal work. What is this licence? It is a formal authority or official permission granted to the applicant that details the rights to perform certain experiments on animals. For example, experimentation requiring animals in the UK is very tightly controlled and requires approval from the Home Office. In fact, it requires three separate licenses granted by the Home Office: (1) Certificate of designation, (2) project licence, and (3) personal licence. What are these licenses?

- *Certificate of designation* The establishment itself, where the regulated experiments involving animals are carried out, must be licensed. It lists all the rooms in the facility where animals may be held, and the procedures that can be carried out there.
- *Project licence* All projects involving animal work must have a licence. This licence is held by the principal investigator.
- *Personal licence* Each person who carries out regulated procedures on animals must also have a licence. They must undergo formal training and are supervised until they are competent to carry out work under the project licence. This licence lasts for a maximum of 5 years.

Each country has its own rules and regulations. We cannot stress enough the importance of understanding and complying with the rules and regulations of the country in which you wish to carry out experiments using animals.

It is your responsibility to know and carry out animal work according to the laws of that country.

Animal Research Facility and Its Staff

A laboratory that holds animals for experimental and diagnostic research is known as an animal facility. This type of facility is also known as an animal house or a vivarium; however, the latter term is used less often now days. A typical animal facility not only holds animals but is also responsible for the daily oversight of animal care.

Employees whose job entails feeding, watering, grooming, cleaning and disinfecting cages, changing bedding, or sterilizing equipment in an animal facility are called animal technicians. Animal technicians, also known as animal-care staff, animal caretakers, animal attendants, or veterinary technologists, may also carry out other duties such as administering prescribed medicines to animals, vaccinating newly admitted animals, recording information regarding an animal's weight, diet, food and water intake, temperature, urine and fecal output, general appearance, etc. Animal technicians work very closely with veterinarians, veterinary surgeons, or informally vets.

Animal research facilities within biomedical institutions are generally located on the top floors or in independent, detached units in order to minimize public access and to prevent unrestricted personnel traffic within the building. The reason for this is to ensure tight security, to reduce allergen and other types of contamination to public areas, and to ensure a calm and quiet environment for the animals. Only animals being used in studies that have been formally approved may be maintained in animal research facility.

Space Description

Animal facilities consist of a number of types of rooms for various purposes. In English, the main types are known as:

- Holding rooms, which contain animals in cages
- Procedure rooms, where specific experiments or studies are carried out
- Service rooms

Holding Rooms

Holding rooms, also known as housing rooms, are rooms where animals are normally kept, either for breeding or stocking. The humidity, pressure, temperature and light-cycles are controlled in this type of room. Based on the length of time that the animals are kept in holding rooms, they can be referred to as *long-term holding rooms* and *short-term holding rooms*.

In addition to the length of stay, the status of a holding room depends on the health status of the animals contained in that room. For instance, health status of rodents in all holding rooms within an animal facility is checked using sentinel rodents. Every holding room contains sentinel rodents, which are primarily used to detect the presence of infectious agents. The number of sentinel animals used in each room depends on the total number of animals in the room. For infection screening, sentinel animals receive dirty material from a portion of other rodent cages in the room during routine cage cleaning for approximately 3–4 months. They are subsequently removed from the room and tested for various common lab-associated mouse viruses such as mouse hepatitis virus (MHV), Sendai virus, mouse parvovirus (MPV), and various parasites such as pinworms and fur mites. Based on the health status of the animals contained in a holding room, they can be also classified as:

- Quarantine/isolation - holding of animals in a separate room for a period of time and until their health status is tested to ensure they are free of disease.
- Clean – animals in this type of room have a clean bill of health.
- Dirty – animals in this type of room have at least one known or suspected disease.

Usage Examples

Animals obtained from non-commercial sources (e.g., universities, research institutions, etc.) must undergo a quarantine period for a minimum of 6–8 weeks and have a negative serological testing result before they can be released from the *quarantine holding room* and placed in a *clean holding room*.

Procedure Rooms

Rooms where experimental manipulations are conducted on animals are called procedure rooms. Each room has its own function and contains equipment for conducting experiments such as lab benches, fume hoods, and biosafety cabinets, among others. Listed below are the English names for the different types of procedure rooms found in a typical animal facility.

- *Surgical rooms* or *operating theatres* are sterile rooms where surgical procedures are carried out.
- *Preparation room, pre-surgical preparation room* or simply a *prep-room*, where the preparation of an animal for surgery takes place.
- *Recovery rooms* or *post-operative recovery rooms* are equipped for the care and observation of animals immediately following surgery.
- *Transgenic room* is the room where foreign DNA, viruses or cells are deliberately inserted into the genome of fertilized animal eggs in order to generate animals carrying the foreign material.

- *Behavioral testing rooms* are experimental rooms used for the study of cognitive processes in animals. These rooms are equipped with various types of mazes, activity boxes, startle response systems, video-tracking systems that record the behavior of animals, among other types of behavioral testing equipment. Behavioral test rooms are generally soundproofed.

Usage Example

The transfer of foreign DNA into single-cell fertilized eggs is carried out in the *transgenic room*; whereas the implantation of these eggs into a surrogate mother is carried out in the *surgical room*.

Service Rooms

Service rooms are also known as support facility rooms. These types of rooms are used primarily by animal-care staff. They include:

- *Feed and bedding storage rooms* provides space to store and protect a limited amount of bulk food for the animals in the facility. The room is designed to protect the bulk food from contamination and infestation.
- *Feed mixing room* is a room for preparing special meals/diets in batches.
- *Cage washing rooms* contains equipment for cleaning cages, racks, water bottles, etc.
- *Cage storage rooms* provide space to store clean cages until needed.
- *Sterilization rooms* contain equipment, such as autoclaves, needed to sterilize items.
- *Waste disposal rooms*, also known as disposal facility, are areas where animal refuse is stored before it is removed from the animal facility. The dead bodies of animals, called carcasses, are stored in a freezer before they are removed from the animal facility.

Since both the animal-care staff and scientists need to work within the facility, it is important that they are able to work without bumping into each other all the time. Therefore, procedure rooms provide the scientific needs for the research staff, whereas the service rooms provide operational needs for the animal-care staff.

Record Keeping

Record keeping is important for good management. It is a requirement and should be carried out according to the rules of the institution and the federal regulations of the country where you work.

Permanent Marking to Identify Individual Animals

It is usually important to be able to identify individual animals in a study. Without identification, it is difficult to keep track of which animals are receiving which treatments or procedures. Animals may be identified using a variety of methods. Listed below are the English names and their descriptions for the different types of methods used to identify animals.

- A distinguishable mark, figure, letter, number, or bars made by puncturing the skin and introducing some ink is called a *tattoo*.
- A metal or plastic identification disk attached to the collar of an animal is a *collar tag*.
- A tiny, rice-sized, electronic device that is implanted under the skin and encoded with a unique and unalterable identification number is a *microchip* (sometimes called a *chip*). This type of permanent marking is "read" by a scanner. The chip transmits the identification number to the scanner, which is then displayed on the screen of the scanner.
- A small plastic or metal object clipped onto the ear is known as an *ear tag*. Ear tags usually carry the individual identification number.
- Clipping off a small tip of the external ear by following an identification chart so that the animal can be identified is known as *ear notching/punching*.
- A metal or plastic identification disk attached to the leg of an animal is a *leg ring*.
- *Toe-clipping*, also known as *toe amputation*, is a method involving the removal of a toe on one or more limbs, following an identification chart. It should be noted that toe clipping may not be widely accepted. Usually, it is only used when no other individual identification method is feasible.

Cage Cards

All animals used in research must be identified, individually or in groups, with cage cards (also known as cage labels). A cage card (or cage label) is a slip of paper used to identify animal(s) in a cage. It contains information about the animal(s) such as supplier, breed or strain, date entry made, investigator's name, project licence number, identification of animals, number of animals, sex, date of birth, etc. Female animals with litters should always have the date of birth of the litter on the cage card. This card is placed on the front of each cage. A sample cage card is shown below:

ANIMAL CODE: P101	DATE: May 10, 2009
PROJECT LICENCE: 9456320M	PI: Dr. A. Frade
SUPPLIER: Jackson Laboratory	CHARGE ACCOUNT: 102407
SPECIES: Mouse	STRAIN: C57BL/6J
SEX: M	# 04
DOB: April 7, 2009	ID#: 36-1 36-2 36-3 36-4

NOTES:
Vasectomised June 24, 2009
TM injection (4 mg/40 g) July 1, 2009
BrdU injection (50mg/kg) July 10, 2009

Definition of terms:

ANIMAL CODE: animal line name
DATE: the date when the mice were placed in the cage
PROJECT LICENCE: is the project licence number
PI: Principal Investigator
SUPPLIER: where the animals came from (source)
CHARGE ACCOUNT: a fund where money is withdrawn to pay for the care of
the animals
SPECIES: Type of animal
STRAIN: a group of organisms of the same species sharing certain traits that are
not shared with other members of the same species.
SEX: Male (M) or Female (F). You can use symbols ($\male, \female$)
#: Number of mice in the cage
DOB: Date of birth
ID#: Identification numbers of the mice in the cage
NOTES: Record information regarding procedures

Data Record Form

A separate data record form should be used to keep tract of individual animals,
their parents, siblings and offspring, tissues obtained from individual animals,
pertinent dates, etc. A data record form contains much more information than
the cage card. Keeping a record of all this is important for good management
and vital to good science. You are responsible to keep the information up-to-
date. Record keeping is a requirement, and records should be kept for a certain
amount of time. For example, records of all procedures carried out on regulated animals must be kept for a period of five years from the time of death or
time released from the establishment. Records are maintained either electroni-
cally or in hard copy. Familiarize yourself with the rules and regulations of the
institution and country you plan to carry out your animal work. A sample data
record form is shown below:

This sample data record form is useful for keeping track of small transgenic animals such as mice and rats.

STRAIN				DATE	
LINE NAME		LITTER #		DOB	
MOTHER		FATHER		GENERATION	
ID#	MARKING	SEX	GENOTYPING ++ +- --	OBSERVATIONS	

Definition of terms:

LINE NAME: the name of the founder and its offspring carrying the particular foreigng ene
LITTER#: A number used to identify the litter
GENERATION: the sequence of generations following the parental generation
MARKING: A distinguishable mark used to identify the individual animals
GENOTYPING: record whether animals carry the specific transgene.
OBSERVATIONS: Record any observable characteristics of the animals

Transgenic Animals

Animals in which their genomes (genetic makeup) have been deliberately modified are called transgenic animals. Generally, transgenic animals carry one or more fragments of foreign DNA in their genomes. The most commonly used techniques to produce transgenic animals are:

- *Pronuclear microinjection* – this technique involves inserting a foreign gene directly into one of the two pronuclei of a single-cell fertilized egg using an ultra-thin glass needle.
- *Blastocyst injection* – this technique involves inserting a foreign gene into embryonic stem (ES) cells, and then inserting the ES cells into blastocysts.

Insertion of a foreign gene anywhere in the genome is known as random gene insertion; whereas, the insertion of a foreign gene at a precise or specific part of the genome is called targeted gene insertion. Pronuclear microinjection results in random gene insertion. Blastocyst injection involves injecting gene-targeted ES cells into 4-day-old blastocysts.

Animals that have been developed from the direct insertion of a foreign gene into its genome are called *founders*. Founders are also referred to as F_0 generation. Founder animals are then mated to establish a transgenic line. Offspring resulting from mating the founder animal are referred to as the F1 (first) generation of animals. Offspring resulting from the mating of the F1 individuals are known as the F2 generation of animals. F1 is the first generation of animals, F2 is the second generation, F3 is the third generation, etc. Blastocyst injection produces animals that contain tissues from both the host embryo and the ES cells. These animals are known as *chimeras*.

Chimera was "a thing of immortal make, not human, lion-fronted and snake behind, a goat in the middle, and snorting out the breath of the terrible flame of bright fire," as Homer described it in the Iliad. In biology, chimera is used to define an animal that has two or more different populations of genetically distinct cells that originated in different zygotes.

Usage Examples

The frequency of *targeted gene insertion* in mouse ES cells increases with increasing amounts of sequence homology.

Targeted gene insertion makes it possible to introduce new genetic information into specific sites on the genome.

Positional effects often occur due to *random gene insertion*.

The lack of precision due to *random gene insertion* may lead to positional effects such as gene silencing.

Administrative Techniques

The act of giving a substance (e.g., medication) by the use of a syringe and needle is called injection. There are several methods of injection. Below is a list of the English names for the most common methods and devices to administer substances into a body, and usage examples.

Injections given just under the skin and into the fat are called *subcutaneous injections* (s.c.), subcut or sub-Q for short.
Injections given directly into a muscle are called *intramuscular injections* (i.m.).

Injections given directly into the blood stream via a vein are called *intravenous injections* (i.v.).

Injections given between the skin layers or just under the top layer of skin are called *intradermal injections* (i.d.). Another name for this type of injection *is intracutaneous injection.*

Injection of a substance into the body cavity is called *intraperitoneal injection* (i.p.).

An injection into the joints is called *intra-articular injection.*

Administering oral fluids into the stomach via a tube is called *gavage.* Gavage does NOT require a needle. It requires a catheter that is passed gently down the esophagus.

Usage Examples

The vaccine was administered by *subcutaneous injection.*

Insulin is administered by *sub-Q injection.*

The clinical dosage of epinephrine given by *intravenous injection* is less than that given by *intramuscular injection.*

Intradermal injection is often used for conducting skin allergy tests.

Mice were anesthetized with *intraperitoneal injection* of 60 mg/kg ketamine.

Intra-articular injection of corticosteroids is an effective treatment of chronic arthritis.

Gavage feeding is a way to feed pups (i.e. young, baby mice) who are not gaining weight because they are not able to suck or swallow.

Management of Stress and Pain in Animals

Both stress and pain can cause suffering in animals. Researchers working with lab animals have an obligation to alleviate unnecessary stress and pain that their experimental animals may experience. This sections aims to give you insight into vocabulary and English usage in this area.

Signs of Stress and Pain in Animals

Animals, of course, cannot tell us how they feel, so it is up to researchers to recognize the signs of pain and stress. In this section we list the signs of stress and pain, and their descriptions.

- Lack of grooming – unkempt appearance
- Activity – animal may be reluctant to move or may be over active
- Eyes may be sunken – eye area does not look healthy, eyes appears deeply recessed

- Piloerection – erection of the hair (hair does not lie down smoothly)
- Excess scratching a particular area – animal scrapes at itself (as to relieve itching)
- Loss of appetite – eats and drinks less
- Vocalization – communicates making sounds (e.g., squeals, cries, or whines when moved)
- Quiet – no vocalization
- Abnormal resting postures – the way an animal holds and positions their body
- Clinical signs – major changes in heart rate, respiration rate, and temperature

Stress and pain are undesirable variables in most research studies. Careful observation of your research animals will tell you whether they are experiencing pain or stress. Please keep in mind that the signs of pain and stress can vary among species, and even among individuals within species. The best way to recognize the signs is to be familiar with the normal and abnormal behavior of the species and individual animals.

Classifications of Drugs to Relieve or Control Pain and Stress

There is some confusion in the terminology surrounding the classification of drugs. Many non-English speakers, including some native English speakers, often misuse or confuse the terms listed below. A brief description for each term is provided to eliminate the confusion or misunderstandings surrounding the definitions.

- Analgesics – are drugs that relieve pain without causing loss of consciousness (e.g. aspirin, Paracetamol)
- Anesthetics – drugs that cause a loss of sensation to pain or awareness. There are two main types: Local and General. Local anesthetics (also known as regional anesthetics) cause a loss of feeling in a specific part of the body without affecting consciousness. General anesthetics put the entire body to sleep; therefore the animal is in a state of total unconsciousness.
- Sedatives are drugs having a calming and relaxing effect. Although, they do not relieve pain but can relieve stress and anxiety. They normally cause drowsiness (a strong desire to fall asleep).
- Tranquilizers are drugs very similar to sedatives; however, they do not cause drowsiness.

Usage Examples

The choice of *local* or *general anesthesia* also depends on the level of pain after surgery.
Sedatives were given to reduce the resistance level of the animal.
Generally, only vets are authorized to handle or administer animal *tranquilizers*.

Humane Methods of Killing

The process of killing an animal with minimum pain and stress is called *humane killing*. There are several methods which are generally considered acceptable.

- Overdose of anaesthetic – an excessive amount of an anaesthetic
- Exposure to CO_2 – inhalation of carbon dioxide (an odorless gas)
- Cervical dislocation – a break in cervical vertebrae (neck bones)
- Decapitation – to separate the head from the body
- Rapid cooling – lowering the body temperature quickly (e.g., on ice)

Overdose of one or more *anaesthetics* is generally used for adult animals of all species.

Exposure to CO_2 in an increasing concentration is generally used to kill rodents and rabbits less than 1.5 kg in weight.

Cervical dislocation must be carried out in a rapid and uninterrupted movement. This method must only be carried out by individuals who are fully trained and competent.

Small foetuses, up to 40 g, can be culled by *decapitation*.

Rapid cooling is generally used for small foetuses belonging to the mouse, rat, or rabbit species.

Be sure to check your local regulations and the project licence on methods that are considered acceptable. Whatever method you decide to use, it is essential to confirm the animal is dead before you dispose of the body.

Ethical Considerations

The use of animals in research is a delicate and complex issue and should not be treated lightly. There has been, and still is, a lot of controversy regarding the use of animals in research. This section is not intended to discuss the ethical arguments for and against animal experimentation; however, we aim to reiterate that English-speaking countries take animal welfare very seriously. All experiments involving animals must be conducted in an ethical way and any procedures carried out on animals must be in strict accordance with the guidelines set out by the country where the experiments will be conducted.

The "3Rs" Principle

All scientists and researchers working with animals should apply the "3Rs" principle – Replacement, Reduction, and Refinement. The 3Rs was formulated by two British scientists, Bill Russell and Rex Burch, in 1959; and is used in many countries around the world. The 3Rs promotes the responsible use of animals in research.

Replacement – avoid using animals whenever it is scientifically possible. Replace animals with computer modeling, established animal cell lines, etc.

Refinement – refine procedures to reduce any discomfort, pain, or distress that an experiment may have caused the animal; and improve animal welfare.

Reduction – reduce the overall number of animals in a study to a minimum without sacrificing the statistical validity of the results.

The use of animals in research is a privilege and should not be abused. Researchers should regard experimental animals as a limited precious resource. All scientists working with animals must treat them as humanely as possible because good animal care is essential to ensure good quality scientific results!

Additional Resources

If your area of work in your new English-speaking lab deals directly with animals, you can find more detailed information about their care and use from the following websites:

www.nc3rs.org.uk/
www.rds-online.org.uk
www.nal.usda.gov/
www.ccac.ca/
www.aalas.org/index.aspx
www.environment.sa.gov.au/animalwelfare/index.html
www.biosecurity.govt.nz/legislation/animal-welfare-act/index.htm
www.lal.org.uk/pdffiles/lafel6.pdf
www.last-ireland.org/
www.frame.org.uk/
http://altweb.jhsph.edu/
http://caat.jhsph.edu/

Unit XV   Latin and Greek Terminology

Introduction

Latin and Greek terminology is another obstacle to be overcome on our way to becoming fluent in medical English. Many English scientific terms come from Latin and Greek. For this reason, romance-language speakers (Spanish, French, Italian, etc.) are undoubtedly at an advantage. This advantage, however, can become a great drawback in terms of pronunciation and, particularly, in the use of the plural forms of Latin and Greek.

Since most Latin words used in medical and scientific English keep the Latin plural ending – e.g., metastasis, *pl.* metastases; viscus, *pl.* viscera – it is essential to understand the basis of plural rules in Latin.

All Latin nouns and adjectives have different endings for each gender (masculine, feminine, or neuter), number (singular or plural), and case – the case is a special ending that reveals the function of the word in a particular sentence. Latin adjectives must correlate with the nouns they modify in case, number, and gender. Although we can barely remember it from our days in high school, there are five different patterns of endings, each one of them is called a declension.

The nominative case indicates the subject of a sentence. The genitive case denotes possession or attachment. Dropping the genitive singular ending gives the base to which the nominative plural ending is added to build the medical English plural form.

For example:

- *Corpus* (nominative singular), *corporis* (genitive singular), *corpora* (nominative plural). This is a third-declension neuter noun that means body. The corresponding forms for the accompanying adjective *callosus* are *callosum*, and *callosa*, respectively. Thus *corpus callosum* (nominative, singular, neuter), *corpora callosa* (nominative, plural, neuter).

Another example:

- *Coxa* var*a* (feminine singular), *coxae* var*ae* (feminine plural), but *genu varum* (neuter, singular), *genua* var*a* (neuter, plural)

R. Ribes et al., *English for Biomedical Scientists*,
DOI: 10.1007/978-3-540-77127-2_15, © Springer-Verlag Berlin Heidelberg 2009

Table 1. The endings of Latin substantives listed by case and declension

Case	Declension							
	1st	2nd		3rd		4th		5th
	Fem.	Masc.	Neut.	Masc./fem.	Neut.	Masc.	Neut.	Fem.
Nominative sing.	-a	-us	-um			-us	-u	-es
Genitive sing.	-ae	-i	-i	-is	-is	-us	-us	-ei
Nominative pl.	-ae	-i	-a	-es	-a	-us	-ua	-es

This unit provides an extensive Latin glossary that includes the singular and plural nominative, and the genitive singular forms of each word as well as the declension and gender of each word. In some terms, additional items have been added, such as English plural endings when widely accepted (e.g., *fetus*, Latin plural *feti*, English plural *fetuses*), and Greek-origin endings kept in some Latin words (e.g., *thorax*, pl. *thoraces*, gen. *thoracos*/*thoracis*: chest)

The endings of Latin substantives listed by case and declension are shown in Table 1.

Examples:

- 1std eclension:
  - Feminine words: *patella* (nom. sing.), *patellae* (gen.), *patellae* (nom. pl). English *patella*.

- 2ndd eclension:
  - Masculine words: *humerus* (nom. sing.), *humeri* (gen.), humeri (nom. pl.). English *humerus*.
  - Neuter words: *interstitium* (nom. sing.), *interstitii* (gen.), *interstitia* (nom. pl.). English *interstice*.

- 3rdd eclension:
  - Masculine or feminine words: *Pars* (nom. sing.), *partis* (gen.), *partes* (nom. pl.). English *part*.
  - Neuter words: *os* (nom. sing.), *oris* (gen.), *ora* (nom. pl.). English *mouth*.

- 4thd eclension:
  - Masculine words: *processus* (nom. sing.), *processus* (gen.), *processus* (nom. pl). English *process*.
  - Neuter words: *cornu* (nom. sing.), *cornus* (gen.), *cornua* (nom. pl.). English *horn*.

- 5thd eclension:
  - Feminine words: *facies* (nom. sing.), *faciei* (gen.), *facies* (nom. pl.). English *face*.

The endings of the adjectives change according to one of these two patterns:

1. Singular: masc. -*us*, fem. -*a*, neut. -*um*. Plural: masc. -*i*, fem. -*ae*, neut. -*a*.
2. Singular: masc. -*is*, fem. -*is*, neut. -*e*. Plural: masc. -*es*, fem. -*es*, neut. -*a*.

Plural Rules

It is far from our intention to replace medical dictionaries and Latin or Greek text books. Conversely, this unit is aimed at giving some tips related to Latin and Greek terminology that can provide a consistent approach to this challenging topic.

Our first piece of advice on this subject is that whenever you write a Latin or Greek word, firstly, check its spelling and, secondly, if the word you want to write is a plural one, never make it up. Although guessing the plural form could be acceptable as an exercise in itself, double-check the word by looking it up in a medical or scientific dictionary.

The following plural rules are useful to at least give us self-confidence in the use of usual Latin or Greek terms such as *metastasis – metastases, pelvis – pelves, bronchus – bronchi*, etc.

Some overseas doctors do think that *metastasis* and *metastases* are equivalent terms, and they are absolutely wrong; the difference between a unique liver metastasis and multiple liver metastases is so obvious that no additional comment is needed.

There are many Latin and Greek words whose singular forms are almost never used as well as Latin and Greek terms whose plural forms are seldom said or written. Let us think, for example, about the singular form of *viscera* (*viscus*). Very few scientists are aware that the liver is a *viscus* whereas the liver and spleen are *viscera*. From a colloquial standpoint this discussion might be considered futile, but those who write papers do know that Latin/Greek terminology is always a nightmare and needs thorough revision, and that terms seldom used on a day-to-day basis have to be properly written in a scientific article. Again, let us consider the plural form of *pelvis* (*pelves*). To talk about several pelves is so rare that many doctors have never wondered what the plural form of pelvis is.

Although there are some exceptions, the following general rules can be helpful with plural terms:

- Words ending in -*us* change to -*i* (2nd declension masculine words):
  - *bronchus* → *bronchi*

- Words ending in -*um* change to -*a* (2nd declension neuter words):
  - *acetabulum* → *acetabula*

- Words ending in -*a* change to -*ae* (1st declension feminine words):
  - *vena* → *venae*

- Words ending in *-ma* change to *-mata* or *-mas* (3rd declension neuter words of Greek origin):
  - *sarcoma* → *sarcomata/sarcomas*
- Words ending in *-is* change to *-es* (3rd declension masculine or feminine words):
  - *metastasis* → *metastases*
- Words ending in *-itis* change to *-itides* (3rd declension masculine or feminine words):
  - *arthritis* → *arthritides*
- Words ending in *-x* change to *-ces* (3rd declension masculine or feminine words):
  - *pneumothorax* → *pneumothoraces*
- Words ending in *-cyx* change to *-cyges* (3rd declension masculine or feminine words):
  - *coccyx* → *coccyges*
- Words ending in *-ion* change to *-ia* (2nd declension neuter words, most of Greek origin):
  - *criterion* → *criteria*

Table 2. List of Latin expressions and abbreviations used in scientific writing

Expression	Abbreviation	Translation
Circa	c. *or* ca.	About (in reference to approximate date or time)
Con fero	c.f.	Compare, consult
Et		And
Et alii	et al.	And others (in reference to people)
Et cetera	etc.	And so forth, and so on
Et sequentes	et seq.	And the following
Exempli gratia	e.g.	For example
Ibidem	Ibid.	The same place
Id est	i.e.	That is
Loco citato	l.c. *or* loc. cit.	At the place already cited
Nota bene	N.B.	Note well (to draw attention to something)
Opere citato	op. cit.	In the work cited
Post scriptum	P.S.	After writing (in reference to additions to a letter after the signature)
Quod vide	q.v.	Which see (in reference to a term/sentence to be looked up elsewhere
Scilicet	sc.	Namely, to wit
Sic	-	As such, thus, so, just as that
Versus	vs.	Against
Videlicet	Viz.	Namely, to wit

List of Latin and Greek Terms and Their Plurals

Abbreviations:

adj.	adjective
Engl.	English
fem.	feminine
gen.	genitive
Gr.	Greek
Lat.	Latin
lit.	literally
m.	muscle
masc.	masculine
neut.	neuter
pl	plural
sing.	singular

A

- **Abdomen**, pl. **abdomina**, gen. **abdominis**. Abdomen. 3rd declension neut.
- **Abducens**, pl. **abducentes**, gen. **abducentis** (from the verb *abduco*, to detach, to lead away)
- **Abductor**, pl. **abductores**, gen. **abductoris** (from the verb *abduco*, to detach, to lead away). 3rd declension masc.
- **Acetabulum**, pl. **acetabula**, gen. **acetabuli**. Cotyle. 2nd declension neut.
- **Acinus**, pl. **acini**, gen. **acini**. Acinus. 2nd declension masc.
- **Adductor**, pl. **adductores**, gen. **adductoris**. Adductor. 3rd declension masc.
- **Aditus**, pl. **aditus**, gen. **aditus**. Entrance to a cavity. 4th declension masc.
  - *Aditus ad antrum, aditus glottidis inferior*, etc.
- **Agendum**, pl. **agenda**, gen. **agendi**. To-do list. 2nd declension neut.
- **Agger**, pl. **aggeres**, gen. **aggeris**. Agger (prominence). 3rd declension masc.
  - *Agger valvae venae, agger nasi, agger perpendicularis*, etc.
- **Ala**, pl. **alae**, gen. **alae**. Wing. 1st declension fem.
- **Alga**, pl. **algae**, gen. **algae**. 1st declension fem.
- **Alveolus**, pl. **alveoli**, gen. **alveoli**. Alveolus (lit. *basin*). 2nd declension masc.
- **Alveus**, pl. **alvei**, gen. **alvei**. Cavity, hollow. 2nd declension masc.
- **Amoeba**, pl. **amoebae**, gen. **amoebae**. Ameba. 1st declension fem.
- **Ampulla**, pl. **ampullae**, gen. **ampullae**. Ampoule, blister. 1st declension fem.
- **Anastomosis**, pl. **anastomoses**, gen. **anastomosis**. Anastomosis. 3rd declension.
- **Angulus**, pl. **anguli**, gen. **anguli**. Angle, apex, corner. 2nd declension neut.
- **Annulus**, pl. **annuli**, gen. **annuli**. Ring. 2nd declension masc.
- **Ansa**, pl. **ansae**, gen. **ansae**. Loop, hook, handle. 1st declension fem.
- **Anterior**, pl. **anteriores**, gen. **anterioris**. Foremost, that is before, former. 3rd declension masc.
- **Antrum**, pl. **antra**, gen. **antri**. Antrum, hollow, cave. 2nd declension neut.
- **Anus**, pl. **ani**, gen. **ani**. Anus (lit. *ring*). 2nd declension masc.
- **Aorta**, pl. **Aortae**, gen. **aortae**. Aorta. 1st declension fem.

- **Apex**, pl. **apices**, gen. **apices**. Apex (top, summit, cap). 3rd declension masc.
- **Aphtha**, pl. **aphthae**, gen. **aphthae**. Aphtha (small ulcer). 1st declension fem.
- **Aponeurosis**, pl. **aponeuroses**, gen. **aponeurosis**. Aponeurosis. 3rd. declension
- **Apophysis**, pl. **apophyses**, gen. **apophysos/apophysis**. Apophysis. 3rd declension fem.
- **Apparatus**, pl. **apparatus**, gen. **apparatus**. Apparatus, system. 4th declension masc.
- **Appendix**, pl. **appendices**, gen. **appendicis**. Appendage. 3rd declension fem.
- **Area**, pl. **areae**, gen. **areae**. Area. 1st declension fem.
- **Areola**, pl. **areolae**, gen. **areolae**. Areola (lit. *little area*). 1st declension fem.
- **Arrector**, pl. **arrectores**, gen. **arrectoris**. Erector, tilt upwards. 3rd declension masc.
- **Arteria**, pl. **arteriae**, gen. **arteriae**. Artery. 1st declension fem.
- **Arteriola**, pl. **arteriolae**, gen. **arteriolae**. Arteriola (small artery). 1st declension fem.
- **Arthritis**, pl. **arthritides**, gen. **arthritidis**. Arthritis. 3rd declension fem.
- **Articularis**, pl. **articulares**, gen. **articularis**. Articular, affecting the joints. 3rd declension masc. (adj.: masc. *articularis*, fem. *articularis*, neut. *articulare*)
- **Articulatio**, pl. **articulationes**, gen. **articulationis**. Joint. 3rd declension fem.
- **Atlas**, pl. **atlantes**, gen. **atlantis**. First cervical vertebra. 3rd declension masc.
- **Atrium**, pl. **atria**, gen. **atrii**. Atrium. 2nd declension neut.
- **Auricula**, pl. **auriculae**, gen. **auriculae**. Auricula (ear flap). 1st declension fem.
- **Auricularis m.**, pl. **auriculares**, gen. **auricularis**. Pertaining to the ear. 3rd declension masc.
- **Auris**, pl. **aures**, gen. **auris**. Ear. 3rd declension fem.
- **Axilla**, pl. **axillae**, gen. **axillae**. Armpit. 1st declension fem.
- **Axis**, pl. **axes**, gen. **axis**. Second cervical vertebra, axis. 3rd declension masc.

B

- **Bacillus**, pl. **bacilli**, gen. **bacilli**. Stick-shape bacterium (lit. *small stick*). 2nd declension masc.
- **Bacterium**, pl. **bacteria**, gen. **bacterii**. Bacterium. 2nd declension neut.
- **Basis**, pl. **bases**, gen. **basis**. Basis, base. 3rd declension fem.
- **Biceps m.**, pl. **bicipites**, gen. **bicipitis**. A muscle with two heads. 3rd declension masc.
  - Biceps + genitive. Biceps *brachii* (*brachium*. Arm)
- **Borborygmus**, pl. **borborygmi**, gen. **borborygmi**. Borborygmus (gastrointestinal sound). 2nd declension masc
- **Brachium**, pl. **brachia**, gen. **brachii**. Arm. 2nd declension neut.
- **Brevis**, pl. **breves**, gen. **brevis**. Short, little, small. 3rd declension masc. (adj.: masc. *brevis*, fem. *brevis*, neut. *breve*)
- **Bronchium**, pl. **bronchia**, gen. **bronchii**. Bronchus. 2nd declension neut.
- **Buccinator m.**, pl. **buccinatores**, gen. **buccinatoris**. Buccinator m. (trumpeter's muscle). 3rd declension masc.
- **Bulla**, pl. **bullae**, gen. **bullae**. Bulla. 1st declension fem.
- **Bursa**, pl. **bursae**, gen. **bursae**. Bursa (bag, pouch). 1st declension fem.

C

- **Caecum**, pl. **caeca**, gen. **caeci**. Blind. 2nd declension neut. (adj.: masc. *caecus*, fem. *caeca*, neut. *caecum*)
- **Calcaneus**, pl. **calcanei**, gen. **calcanei**. Calcaneus (from *calx*, heel). 2nd declension masc.
- **Calculus**, pl. **calculi**, gen. **calculi**. Stone (lit. pebble). 2nd declension masc.
- **Calix**, pl. **calices**, gen. **calicis**. Calix (lit. *cup*, *goblet*). 3rd declension masc.
- **Calx**, pl. **calces**, gen. **calcis**. Heel. 3rd declension masc.
- **Canalis**, pl. **canales**, gen. **canalis**. Channel, conduit. 3rd declension masc.
- **Cancellus**, pl. **cancelli**, gen. **cancelli**. Reticulum, lattice, grid. 2nd declension masc.
- **Cancer**, pl. **cancera**, gen. **canceri**. Cancer. 3rd declension neut.
- **Capillus**, pl. **capilli**, gen. **capilli**. Hair. 2nd declension masc.
- **Capitatus**, pl. **capitati**, gen. **capitati**. Capitate, having or forming a head. 2nd declension masc. (adj.: masc. *capitatus*, fem. *capitata*, neut. *capitatum*)
- **Capitulum**, pl. **capitula**, gen. **capituli**. Head of a structure, condyle. 2nd declension neut.
- **Caput**, pl. **capita**, gen. **capitis**. Head. 3rd declension neut.
- **Carcinoma**, pl. Lat. **carcinomata**, pl. Engl. **carcinomas**, gen. **carcinomatis**. Carcinoma (epithelial cancer). 3rd declension neut.
- **Carina**, pl. **carinae**, gen. **carinae**. Carina (lit. *keel*, *bottom of ship*). 1st declension fem.
- **Cartilago**, pl. **cartilagines**, gen. **cartilaginis**. Cartilage. 3rd declension neut.
- **Cauda**, pl. **caudae**, gen. **caudae**. Tail. 1st declension fem.
  - *Cauda equina* (adj.: masc. *equinus*, fem. *equina*, neut. *equinum*. Concerning horses)
- **Caverna**, pl. **cavernae**, gen. **cavernae**. Cavern. 1st declension fem.
- **Cavitas**, pl. **cavitates**, gen. **cavitatis**. Cavity. 3rd declension fem.
- **Cavum**, pl. **cava**, gen. **cavi**. Cavum (hole, pit, depression). 2nd declension neut.
- **Cella**, pl. **cellae**, gen. **cellae**. Cell (lit. *cellar*, *wine storeroom*). 1st declension fem.
- **Centrum**, pl. **centra**, gen. **centri**. Center. 2nd declension neut.
- **Cerebellum**, pl. **cerebella**, gen. **cerebelli**. Cerebellum. 2nd declension neut.
- **Cerebrum**, pl. **cerebra**, gen. **cerebri**. Brain. 2nd declension neut.
- **Cervix**, pl. **cervices**, gen. **cervicis**. Neck. 3rd declension fem.
- **Chiasma**, pl. **chiasmata**, gen. **chiasmatis/chiasmatos**. Chiasm. 3rd declension neut.
- **Choana**, pl. **choanae**, gen. **choanae**. Choana. 1st declension fem.
  - *Choanae narium*. Posterior opening of the nasal fossae (*naris*, gen. *narium*. Nose)
- **Chorda**, pl. **chordae**, gen. **chordae**. String. 1st declension fem.
  - *Chorda tympani*. A nerve given off from the facial nerve in the facial canal that crosses over the tympanic membrane (*tympanum*, gen. *tympani*. Eardrum)
- **Chorion**, pl. **choria**, gen. **chorii**. Chorion (membrane enclosing the fetus). 2nd declension neut.

- **Cicatrix**, pl. **cicatrices**, gen. **cicatricis**. Scar. 3rd declension fem.
- **Cilium**, pl. **cilia**, gen. **cilii**. Cilium (lit. *upper eyelid*). 2nd declension neut.
- **Cingulum**, pl. **cingula**, gen. **cinguli**. Cingulum (belt-shaped structure, lit. *belt*). 2nd declension neut.
- **Cisterna**, pl. **cisternae**, gen. **cisternae**. Cistern. 1st declension fem.
- **Claustrum**, pl. **claustra**, gen. **claustri**. Claustrum. 2nd declension neut.
- **Clitoris**, pl. **clitorides**, gen. **clitoridis**. Clitoris. 3rd declension
- **Clivus**, pl. **clivi**, gen. **clivi**. Clivus (part of the skull, lit. *slope*). 2nd declension masc.
- **Clostridium**, pl. **clostridia**, gen. **clostridii**. Clostridium (genus of bacteria). 2nd declension neut.
- **Coccus**, pl. **cocci**, gen. **cocci**. Coccus (rounded bacterium, lit. *a scarlet dye*). 2nd declension masc.
- **Coccyx**, pl. **coccyges**, gen. **coccygis**. Coccyx. 3rd declension masc.
- **Cochlea**, pl. **cochleae**, gen. **cochleae**. Cochlea (lit. *snail shell*). 1st declension fem.
- **Collum**, pl. **colla**, gen. **colli**. Neck. 2nd declension neut.
- **Comedo**, pl. **comedones**, gen. **comedonis**. Comedo (a dilated hair follicle filled with keratin). 3rd declension masc.
- **Comunis**, pl. **comunes**, gen. **comunis**. Common. 3rd declension masc. (adj.: masc./fem. *comunis*, neut. *comune*)
- **Concha**, pl. **conchae**, gen. **conchae**. Concha (shell-shaped structure). 1st declension fem.
- **Condyloma**, pl. **condylomata**, gen. **condylomatis**. Condyloma. 3rd declension neut.
  - *Condyloma acuminatum*
- **Conjunctiva**, pl. **conjunctivae**, gen. **conjunctivae**. Conjunctiva. 1st declension fem.
- **Constrictor**, pl. **constrictores**, gen. **constrictoris**. Sphincter. 3rd declension masc.
- **Conus**, pl. **coni**, gen. **coni**. Cone. 2nd declension masc.
  - *Conus medullaris* (from *medulla*, pl. *medullae*, the tapering end of the spinal cord).
- **Cor**, pl. **corda**, gen. **cordis**. Heart. 3rd declension neut.
- **Corium**, pl. **coria**, gen. **corii**. Dermis (lit. *skin*). 2nd declension neut.
- **Cornu**, pl. **Cornua**, gen. **cornus**. Horn. 4th declension neut.
- **Corona**, pl. **coronae**, gen. **coronae**. Corona (lit. *crown*). 1st declension fem.
  - *Corona radiata*, pl. *coronae radiatae*, gen. *coronae radiatae*
- **Corpus**, pl. **corpora**, gen. **corporis**. Body. 3rd declension neut.
  - *Corpus callosum, corpus cavernosum* (penis)
- **Corpusculum**, pl. **corpuscula**, gen. **corpusculi**. Corpuscle. 2nd declension neut.
- **Cortex**, pl. **cortices**, gen. **corticis**. Cortex, outer covering. 3rd declension masc.
- **Coxa**, pl. **coxae**, gen. **coxae**. Hip. 1st declension fem.

- **Cranium**, pl. **crania**, gen. **cranii**. Skull. 2nd declension neut.
- **Crisis**, pl. **crises**, gen. **crisos/crisis**. Crisis. 3rd declension fem.
- **Crista**, pl. **cristae**, gen. **cristae**. Crest. 1st declension fem.
  - *Crista galli* (from *gallus*, pl. *galli*, rooster. The midline process of the ethmoid bone arising from the cribriform plate).
- **Crus**, pl. **crura**, gen. **cruris**. Leg, leg-like structure. 3rd declension neut.
  - *Crura diaphragmatis*
- **Crusta**, pl. **crustae**, gen. **crustae**. Crust, hard surface. 1st declension fem.
- **Crypta**, pl. **cryptae**, gen. **cryptae**. Crypt. 1st declension fem.
- **Cubitus**, pl. **cubiti**, gen. **cubiti**. Ulna (lit. *forearm*). 2nd declension masc.
- **Cubitus**, pl. **cubitus**, gen. **cubitus**. State of lying down. 4th declension masc.
  - *De cubito supino/prono*
- **Culmen**, pl. **culmina**, gen. **culminis**. Peak, top (*culmen*. Top of cerebellar lobe). 3rd declension neut.
- **Cuneiforme**, pl. **cuneiformia**, gen. **cuneiformis**. Wedge-shaped structure. 3rd declension neut. (adj.: masc. *cuneiformis*, fem. *cuneiformis*, neut. *cuneiforme*)

D

- **Datum**, pl. **data**, gen. **dati**. 2nd declension neut.
- **Decussatio**, pl. **decussationes,** gen. **decussationis**. Decussation. 3rd declension fem.
- **Deferens**, pl. **deferentes**, gen. **deferentis**. Spermatic duct (from the verb *defero*, to carry). 3rd declension masc.
- **Dens**, pl. **dentes**, gen. **dentis**. Tooth, pl. Teeth. 3rd declension masc.
- **Dermatitis**, pl. **dermatitides**, gen. **dermatitis**. Dermatitis. 3rd declension.
- **Dermatosis**, pl. **dermatoses**, gen. **dermatosis**. Dermatosis. 3rd declension.
- **Diaphragma**, pl. **diaphragmata**, gen. **diaphragmatis**. Diaphragm. 3rd declension neut.
- **Diaphysis**, pl. **Diaphyses**, gen. **diaphysis**. Shaft. 3rd declension.
- **Diarthrosis**, pl. **diarthroses**, gen. **diarthrosis**. Diarthrosis. 3rd declension.
- **Diastema**, pl. **diastemata**, gen. **diastematis**. Diastema (congenital fissure). 3rd declension.
- **Digastricus m.**, pl. **digastrici**, gen. **digastrici**. Digastric (having two bellies). 2nd declension masc.
- **Digitus**, pl. **digiti**, gen. sing. **digiti**, gen. pl. **digitorum**. Finger. 2nd declension masc.
  - *Extensor digiti minimi, flexor superficialis digitorum*
- **Diverticulum**, pl. **diverticula**, gen. **diverticuli**. Diverticulum. 2nd declension neut.
- **Dorsum**, pl. **dorsa**, gen. **dorsi**. Back. 2nd declension neut.
- **Ductus**, pl. **ductus**, gen. **ductus**. Duct. 4th declension masc.
  - *Ductus arteriosus, ductus deferens*
- **Duodenum**, pl. **duodena**, gen. **duodeni**. Duodenum (lit. *twelve*. The duodenum measures 12 times a finger). 2nd declension neut.

E

- **Ecchymosis**, pl. **ecchymoses**, gen. **ecchymosis**. Ecchymosis. 3rd declension.
- **Effluvium**, pl. **effluvia**, gen. **effluvii**. Effluvium (fall). 2nd declension neut.
- **Encephalitis**, pl. **encephalitides**, gen. **encephalitidis**. Encephalitis. 3rd declension fem.
- **Endocardium**, pl. **endocardia**, gen. **endocardii**. Endocardium. 2nd declension neut.
- **Endometrium**, pl. **endometria**, gen. **endometrii**. Endometrium. 2nd declension neut.
- **Endothelium**, pl. **endothelia**, gen. **endothelii**. Endothelium. 2nd declension neut.
- **Epicondylus**, pl. **epicondyli**, gen. **epicondyli**. Epicondylus. 2nd declension masc.
- **Epidermis**, pl. **epidermides**, gen. **epidermidis**. Epidermis. 3rd declension.
- **Epididymis**, pl. **epididymes**, gen. **epididymis**. Epididymis. 3rd declension.
- **Epiphysis**, pl. **epiphyses**, gen. **epiphysis**. Epiphysis. 3rd declension.
- **Epithelium**, pl. **epithelia**, gen. **epithelii**. Epithelium. 2nd declension neut.
- **Esophagus**, pl. **esophagi**, gen. **esophagi**. Esophagus. 2nd declension masc.
- **Exostosis**, pl. **exostoses**, gen. **exostosis**. Exostosis. 3rd declension.
- **Extensor**, pl. **extensores**, gen. **extensoris**. A muscle the contraction of which stretches out a structure. 3rd declension masc.
  - *Extensor carpi ulnaris m., extensor digitorum communis m., extensor hallucis longus/brevis m.,* etc.
- **Externus**, pl. **externi**, gen. **externi**. External, outward. 2nd declension masc (adj.: masc. *externus*, fem. *externa*, gen. *externum*)

F

- **Facies**, pl. **facies**, gen. **faciei**. Face. 5th declension fem.
- **Falx**, pl. **falces**, gen. **falcis**. Sickle-shaped structure. 3rd declension fem.
  - *Falx cerebrii*
- **Fascia**, pl. **fasciae**, gen. **fasciae**. Fascia. 1st declension fem.
- **Fasciculus**, pl. **fasciculi**, gen. **fasciculi**. Fasciculus. 2nd declension masc.
- **Femur**, pl. **femora**, gen. **femoris**. Femur. 3rd declension neut.
- **Fenestra**, pl. **fenestrae**, gen. **fenestrae**. Window, hole. 1st declension fem.
- **Fetus**, pl. **feti/fetus**, gen. **feti/fetus**. Fetus. 2nd declension masc/4th declension masc.
- **Fibra**, pl. **fibrae**, gen. **fibrae**. Fiber. 1st declension fem.
- **Fibula**, pl. **fibulae**, gen. **fibulae**. Fibula. 1st declension fem.
- **Filamentum**, pl. **filamenta**, gen. **filamentii**. Filament. 2nd declension neut.
- **Filaria**, pl. **filariae**, gen. **filariae**. Filaria. 1st declension fem.
- **Filum**, pl. **fila**, gen. **fili**. Filamentous structure. 2nd declension neut.
  - *Filum terminale*
- **Fimbria**, pl. **fimbriae**, gen. **fimbriae**. Fimbria (lit. *fringe*). 1st declension fem.
- **Fistula**, pl. **fistulae**, gen. **fistulae**. Fistula (lit. *pipe, tube*). 1st declension fem.

- **Flagellum**, pl. **flagella**, gen. **flagelli**. Flagellum (whip-like locomotory organelle). 2nd declension neut.
- **Flexor**, pl. **flexores**, gen. **flexoris**. A muscle whose action flexes a joint. 3rd declension masc.
  - *Flexor carpi radialis/ulnaris mm., flexor pollicis longus/brevis mm.,* etc.
- **Flexura**, pl. **flexurae**, gen. **flexurae**. Flexure, curve, bow. 1st declension fem.
- **Folium**, pl. **folia**, gen. **folii**. Leaf-shaped structure (lit. *leaf*). 2nd declension neut.
- **Folliculus**, pl. **folliculi**, gen. **folliculi**. Follicle. 2nd declension masc.
- **Foramen**, pl. **foramina**, gen. **foraminis**. Foramen, hole. 3rd declension neut.
  - *Foramen rotundum, foramen ovale*
  - *Foramina cribrosa,* pl. (multiple pores in lamina cribrosa)
- **Formula**, pl. **formulae**, gen. **formulae**. Formula. 1st declension fem.
- **Fornix**, pl. **fornices**, gen. **fornicis**. Fornix (arch-shaped structure). 3rd declension masc.
- **Fossa**, pl. **fossae**, gen. **fossae**. Fossa, depression. 1st declension fem.
- **Fovea**, pl. **foveae**, gen. **foveae**. Fovea, depression, pit. 1st declension fem.
- **Frenulum**, pl. **frenula**, gen. **frenuli**. Bridle-like structure. 2nd declension neut.
- **Fungus**, pl. **fungi**, gen. **fungi**. Fungus (lit. *mushroom*). 2nd declension masc.
- **Funiculus**, pl. **funiculi**, gen. **funiculi**. Cord, string. 2nd declension masc.
- **Furfur**, pl. **furfures**, gen. **furfuris**. Dandruff. 3rd declension masc.
- **Furunculus**, pl. **furunculi**, gen. **furunculi**. Furuncle. 2nd declension masc.

G

- **Galea**, pl. **galeae**, gen. **galeae**. Cover, a structure shaped like a helmet (lit. *helmet*). 1st declension fem.
  - *Galea aponeurotica,* pl. *galeae aponeuroticae* (epicranial aponeurosis)
- **Ganglion**, pl. **ganglia**, gen. **ganglii**. Node. 2nd declension masc.
- **Geniculum**, pl. **genicula**, gen. **geniculi**. Geniculum (knee-shaped structure). 2nd declension neut.
- **Geniohyoideus m.**, pl. **geniohyoidei**, gen. **geniohyoidei**. Glenohyoid muscle. 2nd declension masc.
- **Genu**, pl. **genua**, gen. **genus**. Knee. 4th declension neut.
- **Genus**, pl. **genera**, gen. **generis**. Gender. 3rd declension neut.
- **Gestosis**, pl. **gestoses**, gen. **gestosis**. Gestosis (pregnancy impairment). 3rd declension.
- **Gingiva**, pl. **gingivae**, gen. **gingivae**. Gum. 1st declension fem.
- **Glabella**, pl. **glabellae**, gen. **glabellae**. Small lump/mass. 1st declension fem.
- **Glandula**, pl. **glandulae**, gen. **glandulae**. Gland. 1st declension fem.
- **Glans**, pl. **glandes**, gen. **glandis**. Glans (lit. *acorn*). 3rd declension fem.
  - *Glans penis*
- **Globus**, pl. **globi**, gen. **globi**. Globus, round body. 2nd declension masc.
- **Glomerulus**, pl. **glomeruli**, gen. **glomeruli**. Glomerule. 2nd declension masc.

- **Glomus**, pl. **glomera**, gen. **glomeris**. Glomus (ball-shaped body). 3rd declension.
- **Glottis**, pl. **glottides**, gen. **glottidis**. Glottis. 3rd declension.
- **Gluteus m.**, pl. **glutei**, gen. **glutei**. Buttock. 2nd declension masc.
- **Gracilis m.**, pl. **graciles**, gen. **gracilis**. Graceful. 3rd declension masc (adj.: masc. *gracilis*, fem. *gracilis*, neut. *gracile*)
- **Granulatio**, pl. **granulationes**, gen. **granulationis**. Granulation. 3rd declension.
- **Gumma**, pl. **gummata**, gen. **gummatis**. Syphiloma. 3rd declension neut.
- **Gutta**, pl. **guttae**, gen. **guttae**. Gout. 1st declension fem.
- **Gyrus**, pl. **gyri**, gen. **gyri**. Convolution. 2nd declension masc. **Gastrocnemius m.**, pl. **gastrocnemii**, gen. **gastrocnemii**. Calf muscle. 2nd declension masc.

H

- **Hallux**, pl. **halluces**, gen. **hallucis**. First toe. 3rd declension masc.
- **Hamatus**, pl. **hamati**, gen. **hamati**. Hamate bone. 2nd declension masc. (adj.: masc. *hamatus*, fem. *hamata*, neut. *hamatum*. Hooked)
- **Hamulus**, pl. **hamuli**, gen. **hamuli**. Hamulus (lit. *small hook*). 2nd declension masc.
- **Haustrum**, pl. **haustra**, gen. **haustri**. Pouch from the lumen of the colon. 2nd declension neut.
- **Hiatus**, pl. **hiatus**, gen. **hiatus**. Gap, cleft. 4th declension masc.
- **Hilum**, pl. **hila**, gen. **hili**. Hilum (the part of an organ where the neurovascular bundle enters). 2nd declension neut.
- **Hircus**, pl. **hirci**, gen. **hirci**. Hircus (armpit hair, lit. *goat*). 2nd declension masc.
- **Humerus**, pl. **humeri**, gen. **humeri**. Humerus. 2nd declension masc.
- **Humor**, pl. **humores**, gen. **humoris**. Humor, fluid. 3rd declension masc.
- **Hypha**, pl. **hyphae**, gen. **hyphae**. Hypha, tubular cell (lit. Gr. *web*). 1st declension fem.
- **Hypophysis**, pl. **hypophyses**, gen. **hypophysis**. Pituitary gland (lit. *undergrowth*). 3rd declension.
- **Hypothenar**, pl. **hypothenares**, gen. **hypothenaris**. Hypothenar (from Gr. *thenar*, the palm of the hand). 3rd declension.

I

- **Ilium**, pl. **ilia**, gen. **ilii**. Iliac bone. 2nd declension neut.
- **In situ**. In position (from *situs*, pl. *situs*, gen. *situs*, site). 4th declension masc.
- **Incisura**, pl. **incisurae**, gen. **incisurae**. Incisure (from the verb *incido*, cut into). 1st declension fem.
- **Incus**, pl. **incudes**, gen. **incudis**. Incus (lit. *anvil*). 3rd declension fem.
- **Index**, pl. **indices**, gen. **indicis**. Index (second digit, forefinger), guide. 3rd declension masc.
- **Indusium**, pl. **indusia**, gen. **indusii**. Indusium (membrane, amnion). 2nd declension neut.
- **Inferior**, pl. **inferiores**, gen. **inferioris**. Inferior. 3rd declension masc.

- **Infundibulum**, pl. **infundibula**, gen. **infundibuli**. Infundibulum. 2nd declension neut.
- **Insula**, pl. **insulae**, gen. **insulae**. Insula. 1st declension fem.
- **Intermedius**, pl. **intermedii**, gen. **intermedii**. In the middle of. 2nd declension masc. (adj.: masc. *intermedius*, fem. *intermedia*, neut. *intermedium*)
- **Internus**, pl. **interni**, gen. **interni**. Internal. 2nd declension masc. (adj.: masc. *internus*, fem. *interna*, neut. *internum*)
- **Interosseus**, gen. **interossei**, pl. **interossei**. Interosseous. 2nd declension masc. (adj.: masc. *interosseus*, fem. *interossea*, neut. *interosseum*)
- **Intersectio**, pl. **intersectiones**, gen. **intersectionis**. Intersection. 3rd declension fem.
- **Interstitium**, pl. **interstitia**, gen. **interstitii**. Interstice. 2nd declension neut.
- **Intestinum**, pl. **intestina**, gen. **intestini**. Bowel. 2nd declension neut.
- **Iris**, pl. **irides**, gen. **iridis**. Iris. 3rd declension masc.
- **Ischium**, pl. **ischia**, gen. **ischii**. Ischium. 2nd declension neut.
- **Isthmus**, pl. Lat. **isthmi**, pl. Engl. **isthmuses**, gen. **isthmi**. Constriction, narrow passage. 2nd declension masc.

J

- **Jejunum**, pl. **jejuna**, gen. **jejuni**. Jejunum (from Lat. adj. *jejunus*, fasting, empty). 2nd declension neut.
- **Jugular**, pl. **jugulares**, gen. **jugularis**. Jugular vein (lit. relating to the throat, from Lat. *jugulus*, throat). 3rd declension.
- **Junctura**, pl. **juncturae**, gen. **juncturae**. Joint, junction. 1st declension fem.

L

- **Labium**, pl. **labia**, gen. **labii**. Lip. 2nd declension neut.
- **Labrum**, pl. **labra**, gen. **labri**. Rim, edge, lip. 2nd declension neut.
- **Lacuna**, pl. **lacunae**, gen. **lacunae**. Pond, pit, hollow. 1st declension fem.
- **Lamellipodium**, pl. **lamellipodia**, gen. **lamellipodii**. Lamellipodium. 2nd declension neut.
- **Lamina**, pl. **laminae**, gen. **laminae**. Layer. 1st declension fem.
  - *Lamina papyracea, lamina perpendicularis*
- **Larva**, pl. **larvae**, gen. **larvae**. Larva. 1st declension fem.
- **Larynx**, pl. Lat. **larynges**, pl. Engl. **larynxes**, gen. **laryngis**. Larynx. 3rd declension.
- **Lateralis**, pl. **laterales**, gen. **lateralis**. Lateral. 3rd declension masc. (adj.: masc. *lateralis*, fem. *lateralis*, neut. *laterale*)
- **Latissimus**, pl. **latissimi**, gen. **latissimi**. Very wide, the widest. 2nd declension masc. (adj.: masc. *latissimus*, fem. *latissima*, neut. *latissimum*)
- **Latus**, pl. **latera**, gen. **lateris**. Flank. 3rd declension neut.
- **Latus**, pl. **lati**, gen. **lati**. Wide, broad. 2nd declension masc. (adj.: masc. *latus*, fem. *lata*, neut. *latum*)

- **Lemniscus**, pl. **lemnisci**, gen. **lemnisci**. Lemniscus (lit. *ribbon*). 2nd declension masc.
- **Lentigo**, pl. **lentigines**, gen. **lentiginis**. Lentigo (lit. *lentil-shaped spot*). 3rd declension.
- **Levator**, pl. **levatores**, gen. **levatoris**. Lifter (from Lat. verb *levo*, to lift). 3rd declension masc.
- **Lien**, pl. **lienes**, gen. **lienis**. Spleen. 3rd declension masc.
- **Lienculus**, pl. **lienculi**, gen. **lienculi**. Accessory spleen. 2nd declension masc.
- **Ligamentum**, pl. **ligamenta**, gen. **ligamenti**. Ligament. 2nd declension neut.
- **Limbus**, pl. **limbi**, gen. **limbi**. Border, edge. 2nd declension masc.
- **Limen**, pl. **limina**, gen. **liminis**. Threshold. 3rd declension neut.
- **Linea**, pl. **lineae**, gen. **lineae**. Line. 1st declension fem.
- **Lingua**, pl. **linguae**, gen. **linguae**. Tongue. 1st declension fem.
- **Lingualis**, pl. **linguales**, gen. **lingualis**. Relative to the tongue. 3rd declension masc. (adj.: masc. *lingualis*, fem. *lingualis*, neut. *linguale*)
- **Lingula**, pl. **lingulae**, gen. **lingulae**. Lingula (tongue-shaped). 1st declension fem.
- **Liquor**, pl. **liquores**, gen. **liquoris**. Fluid. 3rd declension masc.
- **Lobulus**, pl. **lobuli**, gen. **lobuli**. Lobule. 2nd declension masc.
- **Lobus**, pl. **lobi**, gen. **lobi**. Lobe. 2nd declension masc.
- **Loculus**, pl. **loculi**, gen. **loculi**. Loculus (small chamber). 2nd declension masc.
- **Locus**, pl. **loci**, gen. **loci**. Locus (place, position, point). 2nd declension masc.
- **Longissimus**, pl. **longissimi**, gen. **longissimi**. Very long, the longest. 2nd declension masc. (Adj masc. longissimus, fem. longissima, neut. longissimum)
  - − *Longissimus dorsi/capitis mm.* (long muscle of the back/head)
- **Longus**, pl. **longi**, gen. **longi**. Long. 2nd declension masc. (adj.: masc. *longus*, fem. *longa*, neut. *longum*)
  - − *Longus colli m.* (long muscle of the neck)
- **Lumbar**, pl. **lumbares**, gen. **lumbaris**. Lumbar. 3rd declension.
- **Lumbus**, pl. **lumbi**, gen. **lumbi**. Loin. 2nd declension masc.
- **Lumen**, pl. **lumina**, gen. **luminis**. Lumen. 3rd declension neut.
- **Lunatum**, pl. **lunata**, gen. **lunati**. Lunate bone, crescent-shaped structure. 2nd declension neut. (adj.: masc. *lunatus*, fem. *lunata*, neut. *lunatum*) Lunula, pl. lunulae, gen. lunulae. Lunula. 1st declension fem.
- **Lymphonodus**, pl. **lymphonodi**, gen. **lymphonodi**. Lymph node. 2nd declension masc.

M

- **Macula**, pl. **maculae**, gen. **maculae**. Macula, spot. 1st declension fem.
- **Magnus**, pl. **magni**, gen. **magni**. Large, great. 2nd declension masc. (adj.: masc. *magnus*, fem. *magna*, neut. *magnum*)
- **Major**, pl. **majores**, gen. **majoris**. Greater. 3rd declension masc./fem.
- **Malleollus**, pl. **malleoli**, gen. **malleoli**. Malleollus (lit. *small hammer*). 2nd declension masc.

- **Malleus**, pl. **mallei**, gen. **mallei**. Malleus (lit. *hammer*). 2nd declension masc.
- **Mamilla**, pl. **mamillae**, gen. **mamillae**. Mamilla. 1st declension fem.
- **Mamma**, pl. **mammae**, gen. **mammae**. Breast. 1st declension fem.
- **Mandibula**, pl. **mandibulae**, gen. **mandibulae**. Jaw. 1st declension fem.
- **Mandibular**, pl. **mandibulares**, gen. **mandibularis**. Relative to the jaw. 3rd declension.
- **Manubrium**, pl. **manubria**, gen. **manubrii**. Manubrium (lit. *handle*). 2nd declension neut.
  - − *Manubrium sterni*, pl. *manubria sterna* (superior part of the sternum)
- **Manus**, pl. **manus**, gen. **manus**. Hand. 4th declension fem.
- **Margo**, pl. **margines**, gen. **marginis**. Margin. 3rd declension fem.
- **Matrix**, pl. **matrices**, gen. **matricis**. Matrix (formative portion of a structure, surrounding substance). 3rd declension fem.
- **Maxilla**, pl. **maxillae**, gen. **maxillae**. Maxilla. 1st declension fem.
- **Maximus**, pl. **maximi**, gen. **maximi**. The greatest, the biggest, the largest. 2nd declension masc. (adj.: masc. *maximus*, fem. *maxima*, neut. *maximum*)
- **Meatus**, pl. **meatus**, gen. **meatus**. Meatus, canal. 4th declension masc.
- **Medialis**, pl. **mediales**, gen. **medialis**. Medial. 3rd declension masc./fem. (adj.: masc. *medialis*, fem. *medialis*, neut. *mediale*)
- **Medium**, pl. **media**, gen. **medii**. Substance, culture medium, means. 2nd declension neut.
- **Medulla**, pl. **medullae**, gen. **medullae**. Marrow. 1st declension fem.
  - − *Medulla oblongata* (caudal portion of the brainstem), *medulla spinalis*
- **Membrana**, pl. **membranae**, gen. **membranae**. Membrane. 1st declension fem.
- **Membrum**, pl. **membra**, gen. **membri**. Limb. 2nd declension neut.
- **Meningitis**, pl. **meningitides**, gen. **meningitidis**. Meningitis. 3rd declension fem.
- **Meningococcus**, pl. **meningococci**, gen. **meningococci**. Meningococcus. 2nd declension masc.
- **Meninx**, pl. **meninges**, gen. **meningis**. Meninx. 3rd declension.
- **Meniscus**, pl. **menisci**, gen. **menisci**. Meniscus. 2nd declension masc.
- **Mentum**, pl. **menti**, gen. **menti**. Chin. 2nd declension masc.
- **Mesocardium**, pl. **mesocardia**, gen. **mesocardii**. Mesocardium. 2nd declension neut.
- **Mesothelium**, pl. **mesothelia**, gen. **mesothelii**. Mesothelium. 2nd declension neut.
- **Metacarpus**, pl. **metacarpi**, gen. **metacarpi**. Metacarpus. 2nd declension masc.
- **Metaphysis**, pl. **metaphyses**, gen. **metaphysis**. Metaphysis. 3rd declension.
- **Metastasis**, pl. **metastases**, gen. **metastasis**. Metastasis. 3rd declension
- **Metatarsus**, pl. **metatarsi**, gen. **metatarsi**. Metatarsus. 2nd declension masc.
- **Microvillus**, pl. **microvilli**, gen. **microvilli**. Microvillus (from *villus*, hair). 2nd declension masc.
- **Minimus**, pl. **minimi**, gen. **minimi**. The smallest, the least. 2nd declension masc. (adj,: masc. *minimus*, fem. *minima*, neut. *minimum*)
- **Minor**, pl. **minores**, gen. **minoris**. Lesser. 3rd declension masc.

- **Mitochondrion**, pl. **mitochondria**, gen. **mitochondrium**. Mitochondrion. 3rd declension neut.
- **Mitosis**, pl. **mitoses**, gen. **mitosis**. Mitosis. 3rd declension (from Gr. *mitos*, thread)
- **Mons**, pl. **montes**, gen. **montis**. Mons (lit. *mountain*). 3rd declension masc.
- **Mors**, pl. **mortes**, gen. **mortis**, acc. **mortem**. Death. 3rd declension fem.
- **Mucolipidosis**, pl. **mucolipidoses**, gen. **mucolipidosis**. Mucolipidosis. 3rd declension masc./fem.
- **Mucro**, pl. **mucrones**, gen. **mucronis**. Sharp-tipped structure. 3rd declension masc.
- *Mucro sterni* (sternal xyphoides)
- **Musculus**, pl. **musculi**, gen. **musculi**. Muscle. 2nd declension masc.
- **Mycelium**, pl. **mycelia**, gen. **mycelii**. Mycelium, mass of hyphae. 2nd declension neut.
- **Mycoplasma**, pl. **mycoplasmata**, gen. **mycoplasmatis**. Mycoplasma. 3rd declension neut.
- **Mylohyoideus m.**, pl. **mylohyoidei**, gen. **mylohyoidei**. 2nd declension masc.
- **Myocardium**, pl. **myocardia**, gen. **myocardii**. Myocardium. 2nd declension neut.
- **Myofibrilla**, pl. **myofibrillae**, gen. **myofibrillae**. Myofibrilla. 1st declension fem.
- **Myrinx**, pl. **myringes**, gen. **myringis**. Eardrum. 3rd declension.

N

- **Naris**, pl. **nares**, gen. **naris**. Nostril. 3rd declension fem.
- **Nasus**, pl. **nasi**, gen. **nasi**. Nose. 2nd declension masc.
- **Navicularis**, pl. **naviculares**, gen. **navicularis**. Ship shaped. 3rd declension masc.
- **Nebula**, pl. **nebulae**, gen. **nebulae**. Mist, cloud (corneal nebula. corneal opacity). 1st declension fem.
- **Neisseria**, pl. **neisseriae**, gen. **neisseriae**. Neisseria. 1st declension fem.
- **Nephritis**, pl. **nephritides**, gen. **nephritidis**. Nephritis 3rd declension.
- **Nervus**, pl. **nervi**, gen. **nervi**. Nerve. 2nd declension masc.
- **Neuritis**, pl. **neuritides**, gen. **neuritidis**. Neuritis. 3rd declension.
- **Neurosis**, pl. **neuroses**, gen. **neurosis**. Neurosis. 3rd declension.
- **Nevus**, pl. **nevi**, gen. **nevi**. Nevus (lit. mole on the body, birthmark). 2nd declension masc.
- **Nidus**, pl. **nidi**, gen. **nidi**. Nidus (lit. *nest*). 2nd declension masc.
- **Nodulus**, pl. **noduli**, gen. **noduli**. Nodule (small node, knot). 2nd declension masc.
- **Nucleolus**, pl. **nucleoli**, gen. **nucleoli**. Nucleolus (small nucleus). 2nd declension masc.
- **Nucleus**, pl. **nuclei**, gen. **nuclei**. Nucleus (central part, core, lit. *inside of a nut*). 2nd declension masc.

O

- **Obliquus**, pl. **obliqui**, gen. **obliqui**. Oblique. 2nd declension masc. (adj.: masc. *obliquus*, fem. *obliqua*, neut. *obliquum*)
- **Occiput**, pl. **occipita**, gen. **occipitis**. Occiput (back of the head). 3rd declension neut.
- **Oculentum**, pl. **oculenta**, gen. **oculenti**. Eye ointment. 2nd declension neut.
- **Oculus**, pl. **oculi**, gen. **oculi**. Eye. 2nd declension masc.
- **Oliva**, pl. **olivae**, gen. **olivae**. Rounded elevation (lit. *olive*). 1st declension fem.
- **Omentum**, pl. **omenta**, gen. **omenti**. Peritoneal fold. 2nd declension neut.
- **Oogonium**, pl. **oogonia**, gen. **oogonii**. Oocyte. 2nd declension neut.
- **Operculum**, pl. **opercula**, gen. **operculi**. Operculum, cover (lit. *lesser lid*). 2nd declension neut.
- **Orbicularis m.**, pl. **orbiculares**, gen. **orbicularis**. Muscle encircling a structure. 3rd declension masc. (adj.: masc. *orbicularis*, fem. *orbicularis*, neut. *orbiculare*).
- **Organum**, pl. **organa**, gen. **organi**. Organ. 2nd declension neuter.
- **Orificium**, pl. **orificia**, gen. **orificii**. Opening, orifice. 2nd declension neuter.
- **Os**, pl. **ora**, gen. **oris**. Mouth. 3rd declension neut.
  - Os + genitive case: *os coccyges* (coccygeal bone), *os ischii* (ischium)
- **Os**, pl. **ossa**, gen. **ossis**. Bone. 3rd declension neut.
- **Ossiculum**, pl. **ossicula**, gen. **ossiculi**. Ossicle, small bone. 2nd declension masc.
- **Ostium**, pl. **ostia**, gen. **ostii**. Opening into a tubular organ, entrance. 2nd declension neuter.
- **Ovalis**, pl. **ovales**, gen. **ovalis**. Oval. 3rd declension masc. (adj.: masc. *ovalis*, fem. *ovalis*, neut. *ovale*)
- **Ovarium**, pl. **ovaria**, gen. **ovarii**. Ovary. 2nd declension neut.
- **Ovulum**, pl. **ovula**, gen. **ovuli**. Ovule. 2nd declension neut.

P

- **Palatum**, pl. **palata**, gen. **palati**. Palate. 2nd declension neut.
- **Palma**, pl. **palmae**, gen. **palmae**. Palm. 1st declension fem.
- **Palmaris**, pl. **palmares**, gen. **palmaris**. Relative to the palm of the hand. 3rd declension masc. (adj.: masc. *palmaris*, fem. *palmaris*, neut. *palmare*)
- **Palpebra**, pl. **palpebrae**, gen. **palpebrae**. Eyelid. 1st declension fem.
- **Pancreas**, pl. **pancreates/pancreata**, gen. **pancreatis**. Pancreas. 3rd declension fem./neut.
- **Panniculus**, pl. **panniculi**, gen. **panniculi**. Panniculus (a layer of tissue, from *pannus*, pl. *panni*, cloth). 2nd declension masc.
- **Pannus**, pl. **panni**, gen. **panni**. Pannus (lit. *cloth*). 2nd declension masc.
- **Papilla**, pl. **papillae**, gen. **papillae**. Papilla (lit. *nipple*). 1st declension fem.
- **Paralysis**, pl. **paralyses**, gen. **paralysos/paralysis**. Palsy. 3rd declension fem.
- **Parametrium**, pl. **parametria**, gen. **parametrii**. Parametrium. 2nd declension neut.

- **Paries**, pl. **parietes**, gen. **parietis**. Wall. 3rd declension masc.
- **Pars**, pl. **partes**, gen. **partis**. Part. 3rd declension fem.
- **Patella**, pl. **patellae**, gen. **patellae**. Patella. 1st declension fem.
- **Pectoralis m.**, pl. **pectorales**, gen. **pectoralis**. Pectoralis muscle. 3rd declension masc. (adj.: masc. *pectoralis*, fem. *pectoralis*, neut. *pectorale*)
- **Pectus**, pl. **pectora**, gen. **pectoris**. Chest. 3rd declension neut.
  - − *Pectus excavatum, pectus carinatum*
- **Pediculus**, pl. **pediculi**, gen. **pediculi**. 1. Pedicle. 2. Louse. 2nd declension masc.
- **Pedunculus**, pl. **pedunculi**, gen. **pedunculi**. Pedicle. 2nd declension masc.
- **Pelvis**, pl. **pelves**, gen. **pelvis**. Pelvis. 3rd declension fem.
- **Penis**, pl. **penes**, gen. **penis**. Penis. 3rd declension masc.
- **Perforans**, pl. **perforantes**, gen. **perforantis**. Something which pierces a structure. 3rd declension masc.
- **Pericardium**, pl. **pericardia**, gen. **pericardii**. Pericardium. 2nd declension neut.
- **Perimysium**, pl. **perimysia**, gen. **perimysii**. Perimysium (from Gr. *mysia*, muscle). 2nd declension neut.
- **Perineum**, pl. **perinea**, gen. **perinei**. Perineum. 2nd declension neut.
- **Perineurium**, pl. **perineuria**, gen. **perineurii**. Perineurium (from Gr. *neuron*, nerve). 2nd declension neut.
- **Periodontium**, pl. **periodontia**, gen. **periodontii**. Periodontium (from Gr. *odous*, tooth). 2nd declension neut.
- **Perionychium**, pl. **perionychia**, gen. **perionychii**. Perionychium (from Gr. *onyx*, nail). 2nd declension neut.
- **Periosteum**, pl. **periostea**, gen. **periosteii**. Periosteum (from Gr. *osteon*, bone). 2nd declension neut.
- **Periostosis**, pl. **periostoses**, gen. **periostosis**. Periostosis. 3rd declension.
- **Peritoneum**, pl. **peritonea**, gen. **peritonei**. Peritoneum. 2nd declension neut.
- **Peroneus m.**, pl. **peronei**, gen. **peronei**. Peroneal bone. 2nd declension masc.
- **Pes**, pl. **pedes**, gen. **pedis**. Foot. 3rd declension masc.
- **Petechia**, pl. **petechiae**, gen. **petechiae**. Petechiae (tiny hemorrhagic spots). 1st declension fem.
- **Phalanx**, pl. **phalanges**, gen. **phalangis**. Phalanx (long bones of the digits). 3rd declension fem.
  - − *Os phalangi, pl. ossa phalangium*
- **Phallus**, pl. **phalli**, gen. **phalli**. Phallus, penis. 2nd declension masc.
- **Pharynx**, pl. **pharynges**, gen. **pharyngis**. Pharynx. 3rd declension.
- **Philtrum**, pl. **philtra**, gen. **philtri**. Philtrum. 2nd declension neut.
- **Phimosis**, pl. **phimoses**, gen. **phimosis**. Phimosis. 3rd declension masc.
- **Phlyctena**, pl. **phlyctenae**, gen. **phlyctenae**. Phlyctena (small blister). 1st declension fem.
- **Pia mater**, pl. **piae matres**, gen. **piae matris**. Pia mater (inner meningeal layer of tissue). 1st declension fem. (adj.: masc. *pius*, fem. *pia*, neut. *pium*, tender)

- **Placenta**, pl. **placentae**, gen. **placentae**. Placenta (lit. *cake*). 1st declension fem.
- **Planta**, pl. **plantae**, gen. **plantae**. Plant, sole. 1st declension fem.
- **Plantar**, pl. **plantaria**, gen. **plantaris**. Relating to the sole of the foot. 3rd declension neut.
- **Planum**, pl. **plana**, gen. **plani**. Plane. 2nd declension neut.
- **Platysma m.**, pl. **platysmata**, gen. **platysmatis**. Platysma. 3rd declension neut.
- **Pleura**, pl. **pleurae**, gen. **pleurae**. Pleura. 1st declension fem.
- **Plica**, pl. **plicae**, gen. **plicae**. Fold. 1st declension fem.
- **Pneumoconiosis**, pl. **pneumoconioses**, gen. **pneumoconiosis**. Pneumoconiosis. 3rd declension.
- **Pollex**, pl. **pollices**, gen. **pollicis**. Thumb. 3rd declension masc.
- **Polus**, pl. **poli**, gen. **poli**. Pole. 2nd declension masc.
- **Pons**, pl. **pontes**, gen. **pontis**. Pons (lit. *bridge*). 3rd declension masc.
- **Porta**, pl. **portae**, gen. **portae**. Porta (from Lat. verb *porto*, carry, bring). 1st declension fem.
- **Portio**, pl. **portiones**, gen. **portionis**. Portion. 3rd declension fem.
- **Porus**, pl. **pori**, gen. **pori**. Pore. 2nd declension masc.
- **Posterior**, pl. **posteriores**, gen. **posterioris**. Coming after. 3rd declension.
- **Praeputium**, pl. **praeputia**, gen. **praeputii**. Prepuce, foreskin. 2nd declension neut.
- **Princeps**, pl. **principes**, gen. **principis**. Princeps (first, foremost, leading). 3rd declension masc.
- **Processus**, pl. **processus**, gen. **processus**. Process. 4th declension masc.
- **Profunda**, pl. **profundae**, gen. **profundae**. Deep. 1st declension fem. (adj.: masc. *profundus*, fem. *profunda*, neut. *profundum*)
  - *Vena femoralis profunda*, deep femoral vein
- **Prominentia**, pl. **prominentiae**, gen. **prominentiae**. Prominence. 1st declension fem.
- **Promontorium**, pl. **promontoria**, gen. **promontorii**. Promontorium. 2nd declension neut.
- **Pronator**, pl. **pronatores**, gen. **pronatoris**. A muscle that serves to pronate. 3rd declension masc.
  - *Pronator teres m., pronator quadratus m.*
- **Prophylaxis**, pl. **prophylaxes**, gen. **prophylaxis**. Prophylaxis (from Gr. *prophylasso*, take precaution). 3rd declension.
- **Proprius**, pl. **proprii**, gen. **proprii**. Own. 2nd declension masc. (adj.: masc. *proprius*, fem. *propria*, neut. *proprium*)
- **Prosthesis**, pl. **prostheses**, gen. **prosthesis**. Prosthesis. 3rd declension fem.
- **Psychosis**, pl. **psychoses**, gen. **psychosis**. Psychosis. 3rd declension fem.
- **Ptosis**, pl. **ptoses**, gen. **ptosis**. Ptosis. 3rd declension.
- **Pubes**, pl. **pubes**, gen. **pubis**. Pubis. 3rd declension fem.
- **Pudendum**, pl. **pudenda**, gen. **pudendi**. Relative to the external genitals (lit. *shameful*). 2nd declension neut. (adj.: masc. *pudendus*, fem. *pudenda*, neut. *pudendum*)
- **Puerpera**, pl. **puerperae**, gen. **puerperae**. Puerpera. 1st declension fem.

- **Puerperium**, pl. **puerperia**, gen. **puerperii**. Puerperium. 2nd declension neut.
- **Pulmo**, pl. **pulmones**, gen. **pulmonis**. Lung. 3rd declension masc.
- **Punctata**, pl. **punctatae**, gen. **puctatae**. Pointed. 1st declension fem.
- **Punctum**, pl. **puncta**, gen. **puncti**. Point. 2nd declension neut.
- **Pylorus**, pl. **pylori**, gen. **pylori**. Pylorus. 2nd declension masc.
- **Pyramidalis m.**, pl. **pyramidales**, gen. **pyramidalis**. Pyramidal. 3rd declension masc. (adj.: masc. *pyramidalis*, fem. *pyramidalis*, neut. *pyramidale*)
- **Pyriformis m.**, pl. **pyriformes**, gen. **pyriformis**. Pear-shaped. 3rd declension masc. (adj.: masc. *pyriformis*, fem. *pyriformis*, neut. *pyriforme*)

Q

- **Quadratus**, pl. **quadrati**, gen. **quadrati**. Square. 2nd declension masc. (adj.: masc. *quadratus*, fem. *quadrata*, neut. *quadratum*)
- **Quadrigemina**, pl. **quadrigeminae**, gen. **quadrigeminae**. Fourfold, in four parts. 1st declension fem. (adj.: *quadrigeminus*, fem. *quadrigemina*, neut. *quadrigeminum*)

R

- **Rachis**, pl. Lat. **rachides**, pl. Engl. **rachises**, gen. **rachidis**. Rachis, vertebral column. 3rd declension.
- **Radiatio**, pl. **radiationes**, gen. **radiationis**. Radiation. 3rd declension fem.
- **Radius**, pl. **radii**, gen. **radii**. Radius. 2nd declension masc.
- **Radix**, pl. **radices**, gen. **radicis**. Root, base. 3rd declension fem.
- **Ramus**, pl. **rami**, gen. **rami**. Branch. 2nd declension masc.
- **Receptaculum**, pl. **receptacula**, gen. **receptaculi**. Receptacle, reservoir. 2nd declension neut.
- **Recessus**, pl. **recessus**, gen. **recessus**. Recess. 4th declension masc.
- **Rectus**, pl. **recti**, gen. **recti**. Right, straight (adj.: masc. *rectus*, fem. *recta*, neut. *rectum*)
  - *Rectus abdominis m.*
- **Regio**, pl. **regiones**, gen. **regionis**. Region. 3rd declension fem.
- **Ren**, pl. **renes**, gen. **renis**. Kidney. 3rd declension masc.
- **Rete**, pl. **retia**, gen. **Retis**. Network, net. 3rd declension neut.
  - *Rete mirabilis*
- **Reticulum**, pl. **reticula**, gen. **reticuli**. Reticulum. 2nd declension neut.
- **Retinaculum**, pl. **retinacula**, gen. **retinaculi**. Retinaculum (retaining band or ligament). 2nd declension neut.
- **Rima**, pl. **rimae**, gen. **rima**. Fissure, slit. 1st declension fem.
- **Rostrum**, pl. **rostra**, gen. **rostri**. Rostrum (beak-shaped structure). 2nd declension neut.
- **Rotundum**, pl. **rotunda**, gen. **rotundi**. Round declension (adj.: masc. *rotundus*, fem. *rotunda*, neut. *rotundum*)
  - *Foramen rotundum*, pl. *foramina rotunda*
- **Ruga**, pl. **rugae**, gen. **rugae**. Wrinkle, fold. 1st declension fem.

S

- **Sacculus**, pl. **sacculi**, gen. **sacculi**. Small pouch. 2nd declension masc.
- **Saccus**, pl. **sacci**, gen. **sacci**. Pouch. 2nd declension masc.
- **Sacrum**, pl. **sacra**, gen. **sacri**. Sacral bone (lit. *sacred vessel*). 2nd declension neut.
- **Salpinx**, pl. **salpinges**, gen. **salpingis**. Fallopian tube. 3rd declension.
- **Sartorius m.**, pl. **sartorii**, gen. **sartorii**. Sartorius muscle (tailor's muscle). 2nd declension masc.
- **Scalenus m.**, gen. **scaleni**, pl. **scaleni**. Uneven. 2nd declension masc.
- **Scapula**, pl. **scapulae**, gen. **scapulae**. Scapula, shoulder blade. 1st declension fem.
- **Sclerosis**, pl. **scleroses**, gen. **sclerosis**. Sclerosis . 3rd declension.
- **Scolex**, pl. **scoleces**, gen. **scolecis**. Scolex. 3rd declension.
- **Scotoma**, pl. **scotomata**, gen. **scotomatis**. Scotoma. 3rd declension neut.
- **Scrotum**, pl. **scrota**, gen. **scroti**. Scrotum. 2nd declension neut.
- **Scutulum**, pl. **scutula**, gen. **scutuli**. Scutulum. 2nd declension neut.
- **Scybalum**, pl. **scybala**, gen. **scybali**. Scybalum. 2nd declension neut.
- **Segmentum**, pl. **segmenta**, gen. **segmenti**. Segment. 2nd declension neut.
- **Sella turcica**, pl. **sellae turcicae**, gen. **sellae turcicae**. Turkish chair. 1st declension fem.
- **Semen**, pl. **semina**, gen. **seminis**. Semen. 3rd declension neut.
- **Semimembranosus m.**, pl. **semimembranosi**, gen. **semimembranosi**. 2nd declension masc.
- **Semitendinosus m.**, pl. **semitendinosi**, gen. **semitendinosi**. 2nd declension masc.
- **Sensorium**, pl. **sensoria**, gen. **sensorii**. Sensorium. 2nd declension neut.
- **Sepsis**, pl. **sepses**, gen. **sepsis**. Sepsis. 3rd declension.
- **Septum**, pl. **septa**, gen. **septi**. Septum. 2nd declension neut.
- **Sequela**, pl. **sequelae**, gen. **sequelae**. Sequela. 1st declension fem.
- **Sequestrum**, pl. **sequestra**, gen. **sequestri**. Sequestrum (from sequester, go-between). 2nd declension neut.
- **Serosa**, pl. **serosae**, gen. **serosae**. Serosa. 1st declension fem.
- **Serratus m.**, pl. **serrati**, gen. **serrati**. Serrated, toothed like a saw. 2nd declension masc.
- **Serum**, pl. **sera**, gen. **seri**. Serum (lit. *whey*). 2nd declension neut.
- **Sinciput**, pl. **sincipita**, gen. **sincipitis**. Sinciput. 3rd declension neut.
- **Sinus**, pl. **sinus**, gen. **sinus**. Sinus. 4th declension masc.
- **Soleus m.**, pl. **solei**, gen. **solei**. Soleus. 2nd declension masc.
- **Spatium**, pl. **spatia**, gen. **spatii**. Space. 2nd declension neut.
- **Spectrum**, pl. **spectra**, gen. **spectri**. Spectrum. 2nd declension neut.
- **Sphincter**, pl. Lat. **sphincteres**, pl. Engl. **sphincters**, gen. **sphincteris**. Sphincter. 3rd declension masc.
- **Spiculum**, pl. **spicula**, gen. **spiculi**. Spike (lit. *sting*). 2nd declension neut.
- **Spina**, pl. **spinae**, gen. **spinae**. Spine. 1st declension fem.
- **Splenium**, pl. **splenia**, gen. **splenii**. Splenium. 2nd declension neut.
  - *Splenius capitis/colli mm.*

- **Splenunculus**, pl. **splenunculi**, gen. **splenunculi**. Accessory spleen. 2nd declension masc.
- **Sputum**, pl. **sputa**, gen. **sputi**. Sputum. 2nd declension neut.
- **Squama**, pl. **squamae**, gen. **squamae**. Squama (scale, plate-like structure). 1st declension fem.
- **Stapes**, pl. **stapedes**, gen. **stapedis**. Stapes. 3rd declension masc.
- **Staphylococcus**, pl. **staphylococci**, gen. **staphylococci**. Staphylococcus. 2nd declension masc.
- **Stasis**, pl. **stases**, gen. **stasis**. Stasis. 3rd declension masc.
- **Statoconium**, pl. **statoconia**, gen. **statoconii**. Statoconium. 2nd declension neut.
- **Stenosis**, pl. **stenoses**, gen. **stenosis**. Stenosis. 3rd declension.
- **Stereocilium**, pl. **stereocilia**, gen. **stereocilii**. Stereocilium. 2nd declension neut.
- **Sternocleidomastoideus m.**, pl. **sternocleidomastoidei**, gen. **sternocleidomastoidei**. 2nd declension masc.
- **Sternum**, pl. **sterna**, gen. **sterni**. Sternum. 2nd declension neut.
- **Stigma**, pl. **stigmata**, gen. **stigmatis**. Stigma (mark aiding in diagnosis). 3rd declension neut.
- **Stimulus**, pl. **stimuli**, gen. **stimuli**. Stimulus (lit. *spur*). 2nd declension masc.
- **Stoma**, pl. **stomata**, gen. **stomatis**. Stoma, opening, hole. 3rd declension neut.
- **Stratum**, pl. **strata**, gen. **strati**. Stratum. 2nd declension neut.
- **Stria**, pl. **striae**, gen. **striae**. Fluting, channel. 1st declension fem.
- **Stroma**, pl. **stromata**, gen. **stromatis**. Stroma. 3rd declension neut.
- **Struma**, pl. **strumae**, gen. **strumae**. Struma. 1st declension fem.
- **Subiculum**, pl. **subicula**, gen. **subiculi**. Subiculum. 2nd declension neut.
- **Substantia**, pl. **substantiae**, gen. **substantiae**. Substance. 1st declension fem.
- **Sulcus**, pl. **sulci**, gen. **sulci**. Sulcus. 2nd declension masc.
- **Supercilium**, pl. **supercilia**, gen. **supercilii**. Eyebrow. 2nd declension neut.
- **Superficialis**, pl. **superficiales**, gen. **superficialis**. Superficial. 3rd declension masc. (adj.: masc. *superficialis*, fem. *superficialis*, neut. *superficiale*)
- **Superior**, pl. **superiores**, gen. **superioris**. Higher, upper, greater. 3rd declension.
- **Sustentaculum**, pl. **sustentacula**, gen. **sustentaculi**. Sustentaculum. 2nd declension neut.
- **Sutura**, pl. **suturae**, gen. **suturae**. Suture. 1st declension fem.
- **Symphysis**, pl. **symphyses**, gen. **symphysis**. Symphysis. 3rd declension.
- **Synchondrosis**, pl. **synchondroses**, gen. **synchondrosis**. Synchondrosis. 3rd declension.
- **Syncytium**, pl. **syncytia**, gen. **syncytii**. Syncytium. 2nd declension neut.
- **Syndesmosis**, pl. **syndesmoses**, gen. **syndesmosis**. Syndesmosis. 3rd declension.
- **Synechia**, pl. **synechiae**, gen. **synechiae**. Synechia. 1st declension fem.
- **Syrinx**, pl. **syringes**, gen. **syringis**. Syrinx. 3rd declension.

T

- **Talus,** pl. **tali,** gen. **tali.** Talus. 2nd declension masc.
- **Tarsus,** pl. **tarsi,** gen. **tarsi.** Tarsus. 2nd declension masc.
- **Tectum,** pl. **tecta,** gen. **tecti.** Roof. 2nd declension neut.
- **Tegmen,** pl. **tegmina,** gen. **tegminis.** Roof, covering. 3rd declension neut.
- **Tegmentum,** pl. **tegmenta,** gen. **tegmenti.** Covering. 2nd declension neut.
- **Tela,** pl. **telae,** gen. **telae.** Membrane (lit. *web*). 1st declension fem.
- **Telangiectasis,** pl. **telangiectases,** gen. **telangiectasis.** Telangiectasis. 3rd declension.
- **Temporalis m.,** pl. **temporales,** gen. **temporalis.** 3rd declension masc. (adj.: masc. *temporalis*, fem. *temporalis*, neut. *temporale*)
- **Tenaculum,** pl. **tenacula,** gen. **tenaculi.** Surgical clamp. 2nd declension neut.
- **Tendo,** pl. **tendines,** gen. **tendinis.** Tendon, sinew (from verb *tendo*, stretch). 3rd.
- **Tenia,** pl. **teniae,** gen. **teniae.** Tenia. 1st declension fem.
- **Tensor,** pl. **tensores,** gen. **tensoris.** Something that stretches, that tenses a muscle. 3rd declension masc.
- **Tentorium,** pl. **tentoria,** gen. **tentorii.** Tentorium. 2nd declension neut.
- **Teres,** pl. **teretes,** gen. **teretis.** Round and long. 3rd declension masc.
- **Testis,** pl. **testes,** gen. **testis.** Testicle. 3rd declension masc.
- **Thalamus,** pl. **thalami,** gen. **thalami.** Thalamus (lit. *marriage bed*). 2nd declension masc.
- **Theca,** pl. **thecae,** gen. **thecae.** Theca, envelope (lit. *case, box*). 1st declension fem.
- **Thelium,** pl. **thelia,** gen. **thelii.** Nipple. 2nd declension neut.
- **Thenar,** pl. **thenares,** gen. **thenaris.** Relative to the palm of the hand. 3rd declension neut.
- **Thesis,** pl. **theses,** gen. **thesis.** Thesis. 3rd declension fem.
- **Thorax,** pl. **thoraces,** gen. **thoracos/thoracis.** Chest. 3rd declension masc.
- **Thrombosis,** pl. **thromboses,** gen. **thombosis.** Thrombosis. 3rd declension.
- **Thrombus,** pl. **thrombi,** gen. **thrombi.** Thrombus, clot (from Gr. *thrombos*). 2nd declension masc.
- **Thymus,** pl. **thymi,** gen. **thymi.** Thymus. 2nd declension masc.
- **Tibia,** pl. **tibiae,** gen. **tibiae.** Tibia. 1st declension fem.
- **Tonsilla,** pl. **tonsillae,** gen. **tonsillae.** Tonsil. 1st declension fem.
- **Tophus,** pl. **tophi,** gen. **tophi.** Tophus. 2nd declension masc.
- **Torulus,** pl. **toruli,** gen. **toruli.** Papilla, small elevation. 2nd declension masc.
- **Trabecula,** pl. **trabeculae,** gen. **trabeculae.** Trabecula (supporting bundle of either osseous or fibrous fibers). 1st declension fem.
- **Trachea,** pl. **tracheae,** gen. **tracheae.** Trachea. 1st declension fem.
- **Tractus,** pl. **tractus,** gen. **tractus.** Tract. 4th declension masc.
- **Tragus,** pl. **tragi,** gen. **tragi.** Tragus, hircus. 2nd declension masc.
- **Transversalis,** pl. **transversales,** gen. **transversalis.** Transverse. 3rd declension. (adj.: masc. *transversalis*, fem. *transversalis*, neut. *transversale*)
- **Transversus,** pl. **transversi,** gen. **transversi.** Lying across, from side to side. 2nd declension masc. (adj.: masc. *transversus*, fem. *transversa*, neut. *transversum*)

- **Trapezium**, pl. **trapezia**, gen. **trapezii**. Trapezium bone. 2nd declension neut.
- **Trauma**, pl. **traumata**, gen. **traumatis**. Trauma. 3rd declension neut.
- **Triangularis**, pl. **triangulares**, gen. **triangularis**. Triangular. 3rd declension masc. (adj.: masc. *triangularis*, fem. *triangularis*, neut. *triangulare*)
- **Triceps**, pl. **tricipes**, gen. **tricipis**. Triceps (from *ceps*, pl. *cipes*, gen. *cipis*, headed). 3rd declension masc.
- **Trigonum**, pl. **trigona**, gen. **trigoni**. Trigonum (lit. *triangle*). 2nd declension neut.
- **Triquetrum**, pl. **triquetra**, gen. **triquetri**. Triquetrum, triquetral bone, pyramidal bone. 2nd declension neut. (adj.: masc. *triquetrus*, fem. *triquetra*, neut. *triquetrum*. Three-cornered, triangular)
- **Trochlea**, pl. **trochleae**, gen. **trochleae**. Trochlea (lit. *pulley*). 1st declension fem.
- **Truncus**, pl. **trunci**, gen. **trunci**. Trunk. 2nd declension masc.
- **Tuba**, pl. **tubae**, gen. **tubae**. Tube. 1st declension fem.
- **Tuberculum**, pl. **tubercula**, gen. **tuberculi**. Tuberculum, swelling, protuberance. 2nd declension neut.
- **Tubulus**, pl. **tubuli**, gen. **tubuli**. Tubule. 2nd declension masc.
- **Tunica**, pl. **tunicae**, gen. **tunicae**. Tunic. 1st declension fem.
- **Tylosis**, pl. **tyloses**, gen. **tylosis**. Tylosis (callosity). 3rd declension.
- **Tympanum**, pl. **tympana**, gen. **tympani**. Tympanum, eardrum (lit. *small drum*). 2nd declension neut.

U

- **Ulcus**, pl. **ulcera**, gen. **ulceris**. Ulcer. 3rd declension neut.
- **Ulna**, pl. **ulnae**, gen. **ulnae**. Ulna (lit. *forearm*). 1st declension fem.
- **Umbilicus**, pl. **umbilici**, gen. **umbiculi**. Navel. 2nd declension masc.
- **Uncus**, pl. **unci**, gen. **unci**. Uncus (lit. *hook, clamp*). 2nd declension masc.
- **Unguis**, pl. **ungues**, gen. **unguis**. Nail, claw. 3rd declension masc.
- **Uterus**, pl. **uteri**, gen. **uteri**. Uterus, womb. 2nd declension masc.
- **Utriculus**, pl. **utriculi**, gen. **utriculi**. Utriculus (lit. *wineskin*). 2nd declension masc.
- **Uveitis**, pl. **uveitides**, gen. **uveitidis**. Uveítis. 3rd declension fem.
- **Uvula**, pl. **uvulae**, gen. **uvulae**. Uvula (lit. *small grape*, from *uva*, pl. *uvae*, grape). 1st declension fem.

V

- **Vagina**, pl. **vaginae**, gen. **vaginae**. Vagina, sheath. 1st declension fem.
- **Vaginitis**, pl. **vaginitides**, gen. **vaginitidis**. Vaginitis. 3rd declension fem.
- **Vagus**, pl. **vagi**, gen. **vagi**. Vagus nerve. 2nd declension masc. (adj.: masc. *vagus*, fem. *vaga*, neut. *vagum*. Roving, wandering)
- **Valva**, pl. **valvae**, gen. **valvae**. Leaflet. 1st declension fem.
- **Valvula**, pl. **valvulae**, gen. **valvulae**. Valve. 1st declension fem.
- **Varix**, pl. **varices**, gen. **varicis**. Varix, varicose vein. 3rd declension masc.

- **Vas**, pl. **vasa**, gen. **vasis**. Vessel. 3rd declension neut.
  - − *Vas deferens, vasa recta, vasa vasorum*
- **Vasculum**, pl. **vascula**, gen. **vasculi**. Small vessel. 2nd declension neut.
- **Vastus**, pl. **vasti**, gen. **vasti**. Vast, huge. 2nd declension neut. (adj.: masc. *vastus*, fem. *vasta*, neut. *vasti*)
  - − *Vastus medialis/intermedius/lateralis m.*
- **Vasum**, pl. **vasa**, gen. **vasi**. Vessel. 2nd declension neut.
- **Velum**, pl. **veli**, gen. **veli**. Covering, curtain (lit. *sail*). 2nd declension neut.
- **Vena**, pl. **venae**, gen. **venae**. Vein. 1st declension fem.
  - − *Vena cava*, pl. *venae cavae*, gen. *venae cavae* (from adj. *cavus/a/um*, hollow)
- **Ventriculus**, pl. **ventriculi**, gen. **ventriculi**. Ventricle (lit. *small belly*). 2nd declension masc.
- **Venula**, pl. **venulae**, gen. **venulae**. Venule. 1st declension fem.
- **Vermis**, pl. **vermes**, gen. **vermis**. Worm. 3rd declension masc.
- **Verruca**, pl. **verrucae**, gen. **verrucae**. Wart. 1st declension fem.
- **Vertebra**, pl. **vertebrae**, gen. **vertebrae**. Vertebra. 1st declension fem.
- **Vertex**, pl. **vertices**, gen. **verticis**. Vertex (lit. *peak, top*). 3rd declension masc.
- **Vesica**, pl. **vesicae**, gen. **vesicae**. Bladder. 1st declension fem.
- **Vesicula**, pl. **vesiculae**, gen. **vesiculae**. Vesicle (lit. *lesser bladder*). 1st declension fem.
- **Vestibulum**, pl. **vestibula**, gen. **vestibuli**. Entrance to a cavity. 2nd declension neut.
- **Villus**, pl. **villi**, gen. **villi**. Villus (shaggy hair). 2nd declension masc.
- **Vinculum**, pl. **vincula**, gen. **vinculi**. Band, band-like structure (lit. *chain, bond*). 2nd declension neut.
- **Virus**, pl. Lat. **viri**, pl. Engl. **viruses**, gen. **viri**. Virus. 2nd declension masc.
- **Viscus**, pl. **viscera**, gen. **visceris**. Viscus, internal organ. 3rd declension neut.
- **Vitiligo**, pl. **vitiligines**, gen. **vitiligis**. Vitiligo. 3rd declension masc.
- **Vomer**, pl. **vomeres**, gen. **vomeris**. Vomer bone. 3rd declension masc.
- **Vulva**, pl. **vulvae**, gen. **vulvae**. Vulva. 1st declension fem.

Z

- **Zona**, pl. **zonae**, gen. **zonae**. Zone. 1st declension fem.
- **Zonula**, pl. **zonulae**, gen. **zonulae**. Small zone. 1st declension fem.
- **Zygapophysis**, pl. **zygapophyses**, gen. **zygapophysis**. Vertebral articular apophysis. 3rd declension fem.

UNIT XVI

Unit XVI   Acronyms and Abbreviations

In many fields today abbreviations and acronyms are common. They provide a useful tool for shortening long words or expression in order to save time and space. Some well-known general examples are DVD (digital versatile disc), UNICEF (United Nations International Children's Emergency Fund), NASA (National Aeronautics and Space Administration), and UN (United Nations). Abbreviations are extensively used in the scientific and medical communities. It is common practice to use abbreviations for long names of many clinical diseases and procedures, and for scientific techniques that have to be repeated many times in medical or scientific papers, posters, and oral presentations. This can cause substantial communication difficulties for individuals who are not familiar with English abbreviations in their field. The example below is meaningless to individuals who are not familiar with the abbreviations used.

For example,

> *IHC study of CNS tissue from MS subjects demonstrated loss of PLP-expressing OLs*

Many individuals, including native English speakers, do not know the difference between an acronym and an abbreviation. Acronyms and abbreviations are formed by combining the first letter or letters of several words. All acronyms are abbreviations, but not all abbreviations are acronyms. An acronym is a special type of abbreviation that can be pronounced as a single word (it can be said), while all other abbreviations are pronounced letter by letter (you say each letter individually or spell it out).

For example,

> **AIDS** *is an acronym for* **A**cquired **I**mmune **D**eficiency **S**yndrome *because you say the abbreviation as a word ("aydz"); whereas* **HIV** *is an abbreviation for* **H**uman **I**mmunodeficiency **V**irus *(in this case you say each letter individually).*

It can be extremely frustrating and time-consuming trying to find out what certain commonly used acronyms and abbreviations mean. Abbreviations that some

R. Ribes et al., *English for Biomedical Scientists,*
DOI: 10.1007/978-3-540-77127-2_16, © Springer-Verlag Berlin Heidelberg 2009

consider universally known may be obscure to others. In addition, shortened forms used in one country may not be understood in another. In order to eliminate guesswork and prevent frustration, we have put together an alphabetized list of the most commonly used English acronyms and abbreviations in biomedical research. We feel that having a central reference list at your fingertips could be quite helpful for your scientific communications.

Abbreviation Rules and Style Conventions in English

Apply the following guidelines when using abbreviations:

- On the first occurrence of an abbreviation, spell out the full term, with the abbreviation in brackets. Thereafter the abbreviated form may be used by itself.

  For example,

  Oligodendrocytes (OLs) are the cells responsible for producing a fatty protein called myelin. Each OL can supply myelin for several axons and each axon can be supplied by several OLs.

- Abbreviations may be pluralized by adding an *s* to the end. Plurals of capitalized abbreviations should have no apostrophe because the apostrophe indicates possession. However, plurals of lowercase abbreviations have an apostrophe.

  Examples:

  PCRs (*not* PCR's)
  BACs (*not* BAC's)
  Drs. (*not* Dr's)
  rbc's (*not* rbcs)

  Exception 1: Plurals of some abbreviations, particularly in references, are not formed by merely adding an **s**.

  Examples:

  p for page and pp for pages (*not* ps or pgs)
  l for line and ll for lines (*not* ls)
  c for column and cc for columns (*not* cs)

  Exception 2: Singular and plural units of measure are abbreviated the same. An **s** is generally not added to the plurals.

  1 km and 5 km (*not* 5 kms)

Exception 3: If the abbreviation contains a period (full stop), form the plural with an apostrophe and an **s** ('s). This is probably because it looks more awkward without apostrophes:

For example,

Ph.D.'s
M.D.'s

Exception 4: Plurals of single-letter abbreviations are formed by adding ['s].

For example,

X's

- Abbreviations may be made possessive by adding **'s** for singular possessive, and **s'** for plural possessive.

For example,

EMBO's homepage

- Articles are usually omitted when acronyms are used, being included only when terms or names are written out in full.

Example:

The United Nations International Children's Emergency Fund is a voluntarily funded agency.
UNICEF was created on December 11, 1946.

- The choice of an indefinite article (**a** or **an**) before letter-by-letter abbreviations depends on the pronunciation of the first letter of the abbreviation, not on the written representation of the first letter. If the abbreviation begins with a consonant sound, use **a**. If it begins with a vowel sound, use **an**.

Examples:

an mRNA molecule - although "m" is a consonant, we use the **an** article because the first sound we make is an "em" sound.
an X-ray - this abbreviation begins with a consonant letter, but sounds like it starts with a vowel. The first sound we make is an "eks" sound.

There are several abbreviation styles used today. The only rule one should remember is to have a consistent style.

- Acronyms are generally presented in uppercase letters.

Examples:

AIDS, NATO, BBC, and SARS

However, some acronyms are no longer capitalized. Examples are laser, radar and sonar.

- A period is sometimes written after an abbreviated word (there is no strict rule). The general modern trend is to omit periods from abbreviations (to avoid an appearance of clutter).

Organizations, countries, and units of measure are not generally followed by periods.

Examples:

EU (*not* E.U.)
UN (*not* U.N.)
IBM (*not* I.B.M.)
5 mg (*not* 5 mg.)

Periods are optional with degree titles (this is a matter of preference). However, in modern usage, periods are usually omitted.

Examples where both forms are acceptable:

PhD or Ph.D.
BSc or B.Sc.
MD or M.D.

- If a sentence ends with an abbreviation that requires a period, do not add another period.

For example,

The technician will be here at 4 p.m.
not The technician will be here at 4 p.m.

- Abbreviations of chemicals from the periodic table always start with a capital letter; if there is a second letter, it is always lowercase.

For example,

N   Nitrogen
O   Oxygen
Na   Sodium
Zn   Zinc

- Do not divide abbreviations, or a numerical value followed by a unit of measure, between lines on a page.

.................AIDS   ....10 mg

not..............AI   *not*.................10

DS   mg

Table 1. List of abbreviations and Latin expressions used in scientific writing

Abbreviation	Expression	Translation
c. *or* ca.	Circa	About (in reference to approximate date or time)
c.f.	Con fero	Compare, consult
–	Et	And
et al.	Et alii	And others (in reference to people)
etc.	Et cetera	And so forth, and so on
et seq.	Et sequentes	And the following
e.g.	Exempli gratia	For example
Ibid.	Ibidem	The same place
i.e.	Id est	That is
l.c. *or* loc. cit.	Loco citato	At the place already cited
N.B.	Nota bene	Note well (to draw attention to something)
op. cit.	Opere citato	In the work cited
P.S.	Post scriptum	After writing (in reference to additions to a letter after the signature)
q.v.	Quod vide	Which see (in reference to a term/sentence to be looked up elsewhere
sc.	Scilicet	Namely, to wit
-	Sic	As such, thus, so, just as that
vs.	Versus	Against
Viz.	Videlicet	Namely, to wit

General Abbreviations and Acronyms Used in Biomedical Research

Abbreviation	Definition

A

A	Adenine *or* alanine
aa	Amino acid *or* aminoacyl
Ab	Antibody
ABU	L-a-Aminobutyric acid
ABZ	2-Aminobenzoyl
AC	Accession number
ac	Acetyl
Ac	Actinium
Ac-CO A	Acetyl-coenzyme A
AChE	Acetylcholinesterase

Acm	Acetamidomethyl
ADH	Alcohol dehydrogenase
ADP	Adenosine diphosphate
AFC	7-Amino-4-trifloromethyl-coumaride
Ag	Antigen *or* silver
Aha	7-Aminoheptanoic acid
Al	Aluminum
Ala	Alanine
Am	Americium
AMP	Adenosine monophosphate
Amp	Ampicillin
an	Anisoyl
ANOVA	Analysis of variance
AP	Anteroposterior *or* action potential *or* alkaline phosphatase
APC	Antigen presenting cells
apoE	Apolipoprotein E
APP	Amyloid Precursor Protein
APS	Ammonium persulfate
Ar	Argon
Arg	Arginine
As	Arsenic
ASA	Acetyl salicylic acid
Asn	Asparagine
Asp	Aspartic acid
At	Astatine
ATP	Adenosine 5'- triphosphate
ATPase	Adenosine triphosphatase
Au	gold

B

B	Boron *or* bromouridine
Ba	Barium
BAC	Bacterial artificial chromosome
BAP	Bacterial alkaline phosphatase
BCIP	5-Bromo-4-chloro-3-indolyl phosphate
Be	Beryllium
bh	Benzhydryl
Bh	Bohrium
Bi	Bismuth
Bio-dNTP	Biotin-deoxynucleoside triphosphate
Bk	Berkelium
BLAST	Basic Local Alignment Search Tool
BME	Beta-mercaptoethanol
BMT	Bone marrow (or blood and marrow) transplant
Bp	Base pair

Br	Bromine
BrUrd	Bromouridine
BSA	Bovine serum albumin
bz	Benzoyl
bzy	Benzyl

C

C	Carbon *or* cytosine *or* cysteine
Ca	Calcium
CA	Casamino acids
CAT	Chloramphenicol acetyl
CD	Central domain
Cd	Cadmium
cDNA	Complementary deoxyribonucleic acid
Ce	Cerium
Cf	Californium
CFU	Colony-forming units
CIAP	Calf intestinal alkaline phosphatase
cl	Chloro
Cl	Chlorine
Cm	Curium
Co	Cobalt
Cr	Chromium
Cs	Cesium
CSF	Cerebrospinal fluid
CTP	Cytidine 5'-triphosphate
Cu	Copper
Cyd	Cytidine
Cys	Cysteine

D

D	Aspartic acid
dAMP	Deoxyadenosine monophosphate
dATP	Deoxyadenosine triphosphate
DAG	Diacylglycerol
Db	Dubnium
dCTP	Deoxycytidine triphosphate
ddATP	Dideoxycytidine triphosphate
ddCTP	Dideoxyadenosine triphosphate
ddGTP	Dideoxyguanosine triphosphate
ddNTP	Dideoxynucleoside triphosphate
DEAE	Diethylaminoethyl
DEPC	Diethyl Pyrocarbonate
dGTP	Deoxyguanosine triphosphate
DIDS	4,4'-di-isothiocyanato-2,2'-disulfostilbene

DIG	Digoxigenin
DIV	Days In Vitro
DMF	N,N-Dimethylformamide
DMS	Dimethylsulfide
DMSO	Dimethyl sulfoxide
DMT	Dimethyltryptamine
DNA	Deoxyribonucleic acid
DNase	Deoxyribonuclease
dns	Dansyl
Dnp	2,4-Dinitrophenyl
dNTP	Deoxyribonucleotide triphosphate
DPI	Diphenylene iodonium
Dpr	2,3-Diaminopropionic acid
Ds	Darmstadtium
ds	Double stranded
DT	Diphtheria toxin
DTA	Diphtheria toxin A chain
DTE	Dithienylethene
DTT	Dithiothreitol
dTTP	Deoxythymidine triphosphate
dUTP	Deoxyuridine triphosphate
DV	Dorsoventral
Dy	Dysprosium

E

E	Glutamic acid
EDT	1,2-Ethanedithiol
EDTA	Ethylenediaminetetraacetic acid
EGTA	Ethylene glycol tetraacetic acid
ER	Endoplasmic reticulum
Er	Erbium
Es	Einsteinium
EtBr	Ethidium Bromide
EtOH	Ethanol
Eu	Europium
exo	Exonuclease

F

F	Fluorine *or* phenylalanine
fa	Formylaminoacyl
FBS	Fetal bovine serum
FCS	Fetal calf serum
Fe	Iron
FITC	Fluorescein isothiocyanate

Fm	Fermium
FOA	5-Fluoroacetic acid
Fr	Francium
FSH	Follicle-stimulating hormone

G

g	Gram
g	Gravitational force
G	Glycine
Ga	Gallium
Gd	Gadolinium
Ge	Germanium
GFP	Green Fluorescent Protein
Gln	Glutamine
Glu	Glutamic acid
Gly	Glycine
GM	Genetically Modified
GMO	Genetically Modified Organisms
GUS	Beta-D-glucuronidase

H

H	Hydrogen *or* histidine
Hb	Hemoglobin
HBSS	Hank's Buffered Salt Solution
HCl	Hydrochloric acid
H&E	Hematoxylin and Eosin
He	Helium
HEPES	4-(2-hydroxyethyl)-1-piperazineethanesulfonic acid)
Hf	Hafnium
Hg	Mercury
His	Histidine
HLA	Histocompatibility Leukocyte Antigen
hm	Hydroxymethyl
Ho	Holmium
HPRT	Hypoxanthine phosphoribosyltransferase
HRP	Horseradish peroxidase
Hs	Hassium
Hsp	Heat Shock Protein
HT	High temperature
hU	Dihydrouridine
humi.	Humidity
Hyl	Hydroxylysine
Hyp	Hypoxanthine

I

I	Iodine or isoleucine
Ig	Immunoglobulin
IgA	Immunoglobulin A (gamma A immunoglobulin)
IgD	Immunoglobulin D (gamma D immunoglobulin)
IgE	Immunoglobulin E (gamma E immunoglobulin)
IgG	Immunoglobulin G (gamma G immunoglobulin)
IgM	Immunoglobulin M (gamma M immunoglobulin)
IIe	Isoleucine
In	Indium
Ino	Inosine
IPP	Isopentenyl diphosphate
IPTG	Isopropyl-beta-D-thiogalactopyranoside
IR	Infrared
Ir	Iridium

K

K	Potassium *or* lysine
Kr	Krypton

L

L	Leucine
La	Lanthanum
LB	Luria-Bertani medium *or* Luria broth
Leu	Leucine
Li	Lithium
Lr	Lawrencium
LTA	Lipoteichoic Acid
Lu	Lutetium
Lys	Lysine

M

M	Methionine
mAb	Monoclonal antibodies
MCS	Multiple cloning site
Md	Mendelevium
MeOH	Methanol
Met	Methionine
Mg	Magnesium
MgCl	Magnesium chloride
MMLV	Moloney murine leukemia virus
mmt	Monomethoxytrityl

Mn	Manganese
Mo	Molybdenum
MOPS	4-Morpholinepropanesulfonic acid
mRNA	Messenger Ribonucleic Acid
Mt	Meitnerium
MTS	3-(4,5dimethylthiazol-2-yl)-5-(3-carboxymethozyphe-nyl-2-(4-sulfophenyl)-2H-tetrazolium
mtDNA	Mitochondrial DNA

N

N	asparagine *or* nitrogen
Na	Sodium
NaF	Sodium fluoride
NAD	Nicotinamide adenine dinucleotide
NADH	Nicotinamide adenine dinucleotide (reduced form)
NADP	Nicotinamide adenine dinucleotide phosphate
NADPH	Nicotinamide adenine dinucleotide phosphate (reduced form)
Nb	Niobium
NBT	Nitroblue tetrazolium
Nd	Neodymium
Ne	Neon
Ni	Nickel
NMDA	N-methyl-D-aspartic acid
No	Nobelium
Np	Neptunium
nRNA	Nuclear RNA
NT	Nucleotides *or* nuclear transfer or null type
NTP	Nucleoside triphosphate
NZCYM	Casein hydrolysate casamino acids yeast extract magnesium medium

O

O	Oxygen *or* orotidine
OD	Optical Density
Oilgo(dT)	Oligodeoxythymidylic acid
OMP	Orotidine monophosphate
o/n	Over night
Ord	Orotidine
ORF	Open reading frame
Oro	Orotate
Os	Osmium

P

P	Phosphorus or praline
Pa	Protactinium
PAC	P1 artificial chromosome
Pb	Lead
PBMC	Peripheral blood mononuclear cells
PBS	Phosphate Buffer Saline
Pd	Palladium
PEI	Polyethylenimine
PEG	Polyethylene glycol
PFU	Plaque-forming units
Phe	Phenylalanine
PK	Protein kinase
PIPES	Piperazine-N,N'-bis(2-ethanesulfonic acid)
Pm	Promethium
PMSF	Phenylmethylsulfonyl fluoride
PNK	Polynucleotide kinase
Po	Polonium
Poly(A)	Polyadenylic acid
Poly(A)+	Polyadenylated messenger Ribonucleic Acid
Poly(U)	Polyuridylic acid
Pr	Praseodymium
Pro	Proline
Pt	Platinum
PTX	Pertussis toxin
Pu	Plutonium
Puo	Purine nucleoside
Pur	Purine
PVC	Polyvinyl chloride
Pyd	Pyrimidine nucleoside
Pyr	Pyrimidine

Q

Q	Glutamine or ubiquinone (coenzyme Q)

R

R	Arginine
Ra	Radium
Rb	Rubidium
Re	Rhenium
Rf	Rutherfordium
Rg	Roentgenium
Rh	Rhodium

Rn	Radon
RNA	Ribonucleic acid
RNase	Ribonuclease
RNP	Ribonucleoprotein
RRM	RNA recognition motif
rRNA	Ribosomal ribonucleic acid
RT	Room temperature *or* reverse transcriptase
Ru	Ruthenium
Rxn	Reaction

S

S	Sulphur *or* serine
Sb	Antimony
Sc	Scandium
SDS	Sodium Dodecyl Sulfate
Se	Selenium
Ser	Serine
Sg	Seaborgium
Si	Silicon
Sm	Samarium
Sn	Tin
SR	Sarcoplasmic reticulum
Sr	Strontium
ss	Single stranded
SSC	Sodium citrate buffer
STR	Short tandem repeats

T

T	Threonine
Ta	Tantalum
TAE	Tris-acetate buffer
Taq	Thermus aquatic DNA polymerase
Tb	Terbium
TBE	Tris/Borate/EDTA buffer
TBS	Tris-Buffered Saline
TBST	Tris-Buffered Saline Tween-20
Tc	Technetium
TCA	Trichloroacetic acid
TdT	Terminal deoxynucleotidyl transferase
Te	Tellurium
TE	Tris/EDTA buffer
TEA	Triethanolamine
TEMED	N,N,N′,N′-Tetramethylethylenediamine

TES	N-Tris(hydroxymethyl)methyl-2- minoethanesulfonic acid
Tg	Transgenic
TGB	Tris/Glycine buffer
Th	Thorium
Thr	Threonine
Ti	Titanium
Tl	Thallium
Tm	Thulium
TP	Thymidine phosphorylase
TRIS	Tris-hydroxymethyl-aminomethanel
tRNA	Transfer RNA
Trp	Tryptophan
Tyr	Tyrosine

U

U	Uranium *or* uridine
UP	Uridine phosphorylase
Ura	Uracil
Urd	Uridine
UTP	Uridine triphosphate
UTR	Untranslated region
Uub	Ununbium
Uuh	Ununhexium
Uun	Ununnilium
Uuo	Ununoctium
Uup	Ununpentium
Uuq	Ununquadium
Uus	Ununseptium
Uut	Ununtrium
Uuu	Unununium
UV	Ultraviolet

V

V	Vanadium *or* valine
Val	Valine

W

W	Tungsten *or* tryptophan
WT	Wild-type

X

Xan	Xanthine
Xe	Xenon

X-Gal	5-bromo-4-chloro-3-indolyl-beta-D-galactopyranoside
X-Gluc	5-bromo-4-chloro-3-indolyl-beta-D-glucuronic acid

Y

Y	Yttrium *or* tyrosine
YAC	Yeast Artificial Chromosome
Yb	Ytterbium
YMG	Yeast and malt extract with glucose media
YPD	Yeast extract/peptone/dextrose bacterial media
YPG	Yeast extract/peptone/galactose bacterial media
YT	Yeast extract/tryptone bacterial media

Z

Zn	Zinc
Zr	Zirconium

Please note that amino acids are given three-letter and one-letter abbreviations (e.g. A or Ala for Alanine).

Methods and Techniques Used in Biomedical Research

CHEF	Contour-clamped homogeneous electric field gel electrophoresis
CSGE	Conformation-sensitive gel electrophoresis
DFP	DNA finger printing
DGGE	Denaturing gradient gel electrophoresis
ELISA	Enzyme-linked immunosorbent assay
EMSA	Electrophoresis mobility shift assay
ENDO	Endodeoxyribonuclease assay
EXO	5' and 3' exodeoxyribonuclease assay
FACS	Fluorescence-activated cell sorting
FIGE	Field inversion gel electrophoresis
FISH	Fluorescent in situ hybridization
GC	Gas chromatography
HPLC	High performance liquid chromatography
HTRF	Homogeneous time-resolved fluorescence assay
IEF	Isoelectric focusing
IHC	Immunohistochemistry
IP	Immunoprecipitation
ISH	In situ hybridization
LCR	Ligase chain reaction
MNR	Nuclear magnetic resonance
MS	Mass Spec
MZE	Multiphasic zone electrophoresis

NAAT	Nucleic acid amplification technique
NB	Northern blot
PAGE	Polyacrylamide gel electrophoresis
PCR	Polymerase chain reaction
PFGE	Pulsed-field gel electrophoresis
PRINS	Primed in situ labeling
qPCR	Quantitative PCR
RDA	Representational difference analysis
REMI	Restriction enzyme mediated integration
RFLP	Restriction fragment length polymorphism
RGE	Rotating gel electrophoresis
RPA	Ribonuclease protection assay
SB	Southern blot
SCGE	Single cell gel electrophoresis
SDA	Strand displacement amplification
TAFE	Transverse alternating-field electrophoresis
TAP	Tandem affinity purification
TGGE	Temperature gradient gel electrophoresis
TLC	Thin layer chromatography
WB	Western blot

Radioactive Isotopes

^{14}C	Carbon-14
^{3}H	Tritium-3
^{131}I	Iodine-131
^{32}P	Phosphorus-32
^{33}P	Phosphorus-33
^{35}S	Sulfate-35

Cell Lines

3T3	Mouse embryo fibroblast cell line
9L	Rat glioma
A549	Human lung cancer cell line
B104	Rat neuroblastoma
BHK	Baby hamster kidney cells
B-LCL	B-lymphoblastoid cell line
C6	Rat glioma
CHO	Chinese hamster ovary
CLL	Carcinoma cell line
CMT	Canine mammary tumor

COS	(monkey kidney)
CV-C	African green monkey kidney cell line
EC	Embryonal carcinoma (human)
EJ	Human bladder cancer cell line
GH3	Rat pituitary tumor cell line
HaCaT	Human keratinocyte cell line
HEK	Human embryonic kidney
HeLa	Henrietta Lacks (human cervical cell line)
HL-60	Human leukemia cell line
MCF-7	Human breast cancer cell line
MDCK	Madin-Darby canine kidney
NS0	Mouse myeloma cell line
PC12	Chromaffin cell line (rat)
SCLC	Small cell lung cancer cell line
SPEV	Swine kidney cell line
SW480	Human colon cancer cell line
U87	Human glioblastoma-astrocytoma cell line
U343	Human astrocytoma cell line

Units of Measurement

Always abbreviate units when reporting numerical information. However, if you write the number out in full, you must spell out the unit of measurement. Always put a space between the number and the unit. When starting a sentence with a number and unit, both must be spelled out as words. Abbreviations for most units of measurement use small letters. The following abbreviations of units of measurement are frequently used in biomedical research.

A	Ampere
a	Area
A_{260}	Absorbance measured at 260 nm
Bq	Becquerel
C	Coulomb
°C	Degree Celsius
cal	Calorie
Ci	Curie
cm	Centimeter
cpm	Counts per minute
d	Day
Da	Dalton
DIV	Days in vitro
dpm	Disintegrations per minute
F	Fahrenheit
g, gr	Gram (g is commonly used)

h	Hour
Hz	Hertz
J	Joule
k	Kilo (10^3)
kb	Kilobases
kDa	Kilodalton
L	Liter
lb	Pounds
M	Molar
m	Meter
mA	Milliamps
Mb	Megabase
mg	Milligram
min	Minute
mL	Milliliter
mM	Millimolar
mmol	Millimole
mo	Month
mol	Mole
ms, msec	Milliseconds (ms is generally used)
mV	Millivolt
MW	Molecular weight
N	Newton
n	Nano or sample size
ng	Nanogram
nm	Nanometer
OD	Optical density
oz	Ounces
pH	Power of hydrogen
r	Revolution
rpm	Revolutions per minute
S	Svedberg units
s, sec	Seconds (s is generally used)
T_m	Melting temperature
U	Unit
μ	Micron
μM	Micromolar
μm	Micrometer
w, W	Watt (W is commonly used)
wk	Week
wt	Weight
w/v	Weight to volume
y	Year
V_{max}	Maximum velocity
v/v	Volume to volume

Unit XVII   Conversation Survival Guide

Introduction

Fluency gives self-confidence while its lack undermines you.

The intention of this unit is not to replace conversation guides; on the contrary, we encourage you, according to your level, to use them.

Without including translations, it would have been foolish to write a conversation guide. Why, then, have we written this unit? The aim of the unit is to provide a "survival guide," a basic tool, to be reviewed by upper-intermediate speakers who are actually perfectly able to understand all the usual exchanges, but can have some difficulty in finding natural ways to express themselves in certain unusual situations. For instance, we are strolling with a colleague who wants us to accompany him to a jeweler's to buy a bracelet for his wife. Bear in mind that, even in your own language, fluency is virtually impossible in all situations. I have only been upset and disappointed (in English) three times. At a laundry, at an airport, and, on a third occasion, at a restaurant. I had considered myself relatively fluent in English up to that time, but, under pressure, thoughts come to mind much faster than words and your level of fluency can be overwhelmed as a consequence of the adrenaline levels in your blood. Accept the following piece of advice: unless you are bilingual, you cannot afford to get into arguments in a language other than your own.

Many upper-intermediate speakers do not take a conversation guide when traveling abroad. They think their level is well above those who need a guide to construct basic sentences and are ashamed of being seen reading one (I myself went through this stage). I was (and they are) utterly wrong in not taking a guide because, for upper-intermediate speakers, a conversation guide has different and very important uses (as my level increased, I realized that my use of these guides changed; I did not need to read the translations, except for a few words, and I just looked for natural ways of saying things).

In my opinion, even for those who are bilingual, conversation guides are extremely helpful whenever you are in an unfamiliar environment such as, for example, a florist. How many names of flowers do you know in your own language? Probably fewer than a dozen. Think that every conversation scenario has its own jargon and a conversation guide can give you the hints that an upper-intermediate speaker may need to be actually fluent in many situations.

R. Ribes et al., *English for Biomedical Scientists*,
DOI: 10.1007/978-3-540-77127-2_17, © Springer-Verlag Berlin Heidelberg 2009

So, do not be ashamed of carrying and reading a guide, even in public; they are the shortest way to fluency in those unfamiliar situations that sporadically test our English level and, more importantly, our self-confidence in English.

Whenever you have to go out for dinner, for example, review the key words and usual sentences of your conversation guide. It will not take more than ten minutes, and your dinner will taste even better since you have ordered it with unbelievable fluency and precision. What is just a recommendable task for upper-intermediate speakers is absolutely mandatory for lower-intermediate speakers who, before leaving the hotel, should review and rehearse the sentences they will need to ask for whatever they want to eat or, at least, to avoid ordering what they never would eat in their own country. Looking at the faces of your colleagues once the first course is served, you will realize who is eating what he wanted and who, in contrast, does not know what he ordered and, what is worse, what he is actually eating.

Let us think for a moment about the incident that happened to me when I was at UCSF Medical Center. I was invited to have lunch at a diner near the hospital, and when I asked for still mineral water, the somewhat surprised waiter answered that they did not have still mineral water but sparkling, because no customer had ever asked for such a "delicacy," and offered me plain water instead. (If you do not understand this story, the important words to look up in the dictionary are "diner", with one "n", "still", "sparkling," and "plain.")

Would you be fluent without the help of a guide in a car breakdown? I actually had a leaky gas tank on a trip with my wife and mother-in-law from Boston to Niagara Falls and Toronto. I still remember the face of the mechanic in Toronto when asking me if we were staying in downtown Toronto. I answered that we were on our way back to … Boston. I can tell you that my worn guide was vital; without it, I would not have been able to explain what the problem was. This was the last time I had to take the guide from a hidden pocket in my suitcase. Since then I have kept my guide with me, even at … the beach, because unexpected situations may arise at any time by definition. Think of possibly embarrassing, although not infrequent, situations and … do not forget your guide on your next trip abroad (the inside pocket of your jacket is a suitable place for those who still have not overcome the stage of "guide-ashamedness").

Those who have reached a certain level are aware of the many embarrassing situations they have had to overcome in the past to become fluent in a majority of circumstances.

Greetings

- Hi.
- Hello.
- Good morning.
- Good afternoon.
- Good evening.

- Good night.
- How are you? (Very) Well, thank you.
- How are you getting on? All right, thank you.
- I am glad to see you.
- Nice to see you (again).
- How do you feel today?
- How is your family?

- Good-bye.
- Bye-bye.
- See you later.
- See you soon.
- See you tomorrow.
- Give my regards to everybody.
- Give my love to your children.

Presentations

- This is Mr./Mrs. …
- These are Mister and Missus …
- My name is …
- What is your name? My name is …
- Pleased/Nice to meet you.
- Let me introduce you to …
- I'd like to introduce you to …
- Have you already met Mr. …? Yes, I have.

Personal Data

- What is your name? My name is …
- What is your surname/family name? My surname/family name is …
- Where are you from? I am from …
- Where do you live? I live in …
- What is your address? My address is …
- What is your email address? My email address is …
- What is your phone number? My phone number is …
- What is your mobile phone/cellular number? My mobile phone/cellular number is …
- How old are you? I am …
- Where were you born? I was born in …
- What do you do? I am a scientist.
- What do you do? I do research on …

Courtesy Sentences

- Thank you very much. You are welcome (don't mention it).
- Would you please ...? Sure, it is a pleasure.
- Excusem e.
- Pardon.
- Sorry.
- Cheers!
- Congratulations!
- Good luck!
- It doesn't matter!
- May I help you?
- Here you are?
- You are very kind. It is very kind of you.
- Don't worry, that's not what I wanted.
- Sorry to bother/trouble you.
- Don't worry!
- What can I do for you?
- How can I help you?
- Would you like something to drink?
- Would you like a cigarette?
- I would like ...
- I beg your pardon.
- Have a nice day.

Speaking in a Foreign Language

- Do you speak English/Spanish/French ...? I do not speak English/Only a bit/Not a word.
- Do you understand me? Yes, I do. No, I don't.
- Sorry, I do not understand you.
- Could you speak slowly, please?
- How do you write it?
- Could you write it down?
- How do you spell it?
- How do you pronounce it?
- Sorry, what did you say?
- Sorry, my English is not very good.
- Sorry, I didn't get that.
- Could you please repeat that?
- I can't hear you.

At the Restaurant

"The same for me" is one of the most common sentences heard at tables around the world. The non-fluent English speaker links his/her gastronomic fate to a reportedly more fluent one in order to avoid uncomfortable counter-questions such as "How would you like your meat, sir?"

A simple look at a guide a few minutes before the dinner will provide you with enough vocabulary to ask for whatever you want.

Do not let your lack of fluency spoil a good opportunity to taste delicious dishes or wines.

Preliminary Exchanges

- Hello, have you got a table for three people?
- Hi, may I book a table for a party of seven at 6 o'clock?
- What time are you coming, sir?
- Where can we sit?
- Is this chair free?
- Is this table taken?
- Waiter/waitress, I would like to order.
- Could I see the menu?
- Could you bring the menu?
- Can I have the wine list?
- Could you give us a table next to the window?
- Could you give me a table on the mezzanine?
- Could you give us a table near the stage?

Ordering

- We'd like to order now.
- Could you bring us some bread, please?
- We'd like to have something to drink.
- Here you are.
- Could you recommend a local wine?
- Could you recommend one of your specialties?
- Could you suggest something special?
- What are the ingredients of this dish?
- I'll have a steamed lobster, please.
- How would you like your meat, sir?
- Rare/medium-rare/medium/well-done.
- Somewhere between rare and medium rare will be OK.
- Is the halibut fresh?

- What is there for dessert?
- Anything else, sir?
- No, we are fine, thank you.
- The same for me.
- Enjoy your meal, sir.
- How was everything, sir?
- The meal was excellent.
- The sirloin was delicious.
- Excuse me, I have spilt something on my tie. Could you help me?

Complaining

- The dish is cold. Would you please heat it up?
- The meat is underdone. Would you cook it a little more, please?
- Excuse me. This is not what I asked for.
- Could you change this for me?
- The fish is not fresh. I want to see the manager.
- I asked for a sirloin.
- The meal wasn't very good.
- The meat smells off.
- Could you bring the complaints book?
- This wine is off, I think …
- Waiter,t his fork is dirty.

The Check (*UK*, The *Bill*)

- The check, please
- Would you bring us the check, please?
- All together, please.
- We are paying separately.
- I am afraid there is a mistake, we didn't have this.
- This is for you.
- Keep the change.

City Transportation

- I want to go to the Metropolitan museum.
- Which bus/tram/underground line must I take for the Metropolitan?
- Which bus/tram/underground line can I take to get to the Metropolitan?
- Where does the number … bus stop?
- Does this bus go to …?
- How much is a single ticket?

- Three tickets, please.
- Where must I get off for …?
- Is this seat occupied/vacant?
- Where can I get a taxi?
- How much is the fare for …?
- Take me to … Street.
- Do you know where the … is?

Shopping

Asking About Store Hours

- When are you open?
- How late are you open today?
- Are you open on Saturday?

Preliminary Exchanges

- Hello sir (madam), may I help you?
- Can I help you find something?
- Thank you, I am just looking.
- I just can't make up my mind.
- Can I help you with something?
- If I can help you, just let me know.
- Are you looking for something in particular?
- I am looking for something for my wife.
- I am looking for something for my husband.
- I am looking for something for my children.
- It is a gift.
- Hi, do you sell …?
- I am looking for a … Can you help me?
- Would you tell me where the music department is?
- Which floor is the leather goods department on? On the ground floor (on the mezzanine, on the second floor …)
- Please would you show me …?
- What kind do you want?
- Where can I find the mirror? There is a mirror over there.
- The changing rooms are over there.
- Only four items are allowed in the dressing room at a time.
- Is there a public rest room here?
- Have you decided?
- Have you made up your mind?

Buying Clothes/Shoes

- Please can you show me some natural silk ties?
- I want to buy a long-sleeved shirt.
- I want the pair of high-heeled shoes I have seen in the window.
- Would you please show me the pair in the window?
- What material is it?
- What material is it made of? Cotton, leather, linen, wool, velvet, silk, nylon, acrylic fiber.
- What size, please?
- What size do you need?
- Is this my size?
- Do you think this is my size?
- Where is the fitting room?
- Does it fit you?
- I think it fits well, although the collar is a little tight.
- No, it doesn't fit me.
- May I try a larger size?
- I'll try a smaller size. Would you mind bringing it to me?
- I'll take this one.
- How much is it?
- This is too expensive.
- Oh, this is a bargain!
- I like it.
- May I try this on?
- In which color? Navy blue, please.
- Do you have anything to go with this?
- I need a belt/a pair of socks/pair of jeans/pair of gloves ...
- I need a size 38.
- I don't know my size. Can you measure me?
- Would you measure my waist, please?
- Do you have a shirt to match this?
- Do you have this in blue/in wool/in a larger size/in a smaller size?
- Do you have something a bit less expensive?
- I'd like to try this on. Where is the fitting room?
- How would you like to pay for this? Cash/credit.
- We don't have that in your size/color.
- We are out of that item.
- It's too tight/loose.
- It's too expensive/cheap.
- I don't like the color.
- Is it on sale?
- Can I have this gift wrapped?

At the Shoe Shop

- A pair of shoes, boots, sandals, slippers ..., shoelace, sole, heel, leather, suede, rubber, shoehorn.
- What kind of shoes do you want?
- I want a pair of rubber-soled shoes/high-heeled shoes/leather shoes/suede slippers/boots.
- I want a pair of lace-up/slip-on shoes good for the rain/for walking.
- What is your size, please?
- They are a little tight/too large/too small.
- Would you please show me the pair in the window?
- Can I try a smaller/larger size, please?
- This one fits well.
- I would like some shoe polish.
- I need some new laces
- I need a shoe-horn.

At the Post Office

- I need some (first class) stamps, please.
- First class, please.
- Air mail, please.
- I would like this to go express mail.
- I would like this recorded/special delivery.
- I need to send this second-day mail (US).
- Second-class for this, please (UK).
- I need to send this parcel post.
- I need to send this by certified mail.
- I need to send this by registered mail.
- Return receipt requested, please.
- How much postage do I need for this?
- How much postage do I need to send this air mail?
- Do you have any envelopes?
- How long will it take to get there? It should arrive on Monday.
- The forms are over there. Please fill out (UK, fill in) a form and bring it back to me.

Going to the Theater (*UK*, Theatre)

- Sorry, we are sold out tonight.
- Sorry, these tickets are non-refundable.

- Sorry, there are no tickets available.
- Would you like to make a reservation for another night?
- I would like two seats for tonight's performance, please.
- Where are the best seats you have left?
- Do you have anything in the first four rows?
- Do you have matinees?
- How much are the tickets?
- Is it possible to exchange these for another night?
- Do you take a check/credit cards?
- How long does the show run? About two hours.
- When does the show close?
- Is there an intermission? There is an intermission.
- Where are the rest rooms?
- Where is the cloakroom?
- Is there anywhere we can leave our coats?
- Do you sell concessions?
- How soon does the curtain go up?
- Did you make a reservation?
- What name did you reserve the tickets under?
- The usher will give you your program (*UK*, programme).

At the Drugstore (*UK*, Chemist)

- Prescription, tablet, pill, cream, suppository, laxative, sedative, injection, bandage, sticking plasters, cotton wool, gauze, alcohol, thermometer, sanitary towels, napkins, toothpaste, toothbrush, paper tissues, duty chemist.
- Fever, cold, cough, headache, toothache, diarrhea, constipation, sickness, insomnia, sunburn, insect bite.
- I am looking for something for ...
- Could you give me ...?
- Could you give me something for ...?
- I need some aspirin/antiseptic/eye drops/foot powder.
- I need razor blades and shaving cream.
- What are the side effects of this drug?
- Will this make me drowsy?
- Should I take this with meals?

At the Cosmetics Counter

- Soap, shampoo, deodorant, shower gel, hair spray, sun tan cream, comb, hairbrush, toothpaste, toothbrush, make-up, cologne, lipstick, perfume, hair remover, scissors, face lotion, cleansing cream, razor, shaving foam.

At the Bookshop/Newsagent's

- I would like to buy a book on the history of the city.
- Has this book been translated into Japanese?
- Have you got Swedish newspapers/magazines/books?
- Where can I buy a road map?

At the Photography Shop

- I want a 36-exposure film for this camera.
- I want new batteries for my camera.
- Could you develop this film?
- Could you develop this film with two prints of each photograph?
- How much does developing cost?
- When will the photographs be ready?
- My camera is not working, would you have a look at it?
- Do you take passport (ID) photographs?
- I want an enlargement of this one and two copies of this other.
- Have you got a 64-megabyte data card to fit this camera?
- How much would a 128-megabyte card be?
- How many megapixels is this one?
- Has it got an optical zoom?
- Can you print the pictures on this CD?

At the Florist

- I would like to order a bouquet of roses.
- You can choose violets and orchids in several colors.
- Which flowers are the freshest?
- What are these flowers called?
- Do you deliver?
- Could you please send this bouquet to the NH Abascal hotel manager at 47 Abascal St. before noon?
- Could you please send this card too?

Paying

- Where is the cash machine (or ATM machine)?
- Is there a cashpoint near here?
- How much is that all together?
- Will you pay cash or by credit card?

- Next in line (queue).
- Could you gift-wrap it for me?
- Can I have a receipt, please?
- Is there a cashpoint near here?

At the Hairdresser

When I was in Boston I went to a hairdresser's and my lack of fluency was responsible for a drastic change in my image for a couple of months so that my wife almost did not recognize me when I picked her up at Logan on one of her multiple visits to New England. I can assure you that I will never forget the word "sideburns"; the hairdresser, a robust Afro-American lady, drastically cut them before I could recall the name of this insignificant part of my facial hair. To tell you the truth, I did not know how important sideburns were until I didn't have them.

If you do not trust an unknown hairdresser, "just a trim" would be a polite way of avoiding a disaster.

I recommend, before going to the hairdresser, a thorough review of your guide so that you get familiar with key words such as: scissors, comb, brush, dryer, shampooing, hair style, hair cut, manicure, dyeing, shave, beard, moustache, sideburns (!), fringe, curl, or plait.

Men and Women

- How long will I have to wait?
- Is the water OK? It is fine/too hot/too cold.
- My hair is greasy/dry.
- I have dandruff.
- I am losing a lot of hair.
- A shampoo and rinse, please.
- How would you like it?
- Are you going for a particular look?
- I want a (hair) cut like this.
- Just a trim, please.
- However you want.
- Is it OK?
- That's fine, thank you.
- How much is it?
- How much do I owe you?
- Do you do highlights?
- I would like a tint, please.

Men

- I want a shave.
- A razor cut, please.
- Just a trim, please.
- Leave the sideburns as they are (!).
- Trim the moustache.
- Trim my beard and moustache, please.
- Towards the back, without any parting.
- I part my hair on the left/in the middle.
- Leave it long.
- Could you take a little more off the top/the back/the sides?
- How much do you want me to take off?

Women

- How do I set your hair?
- What hair style do you want?
- I would like my hair dyed.
- Same color?
- A little darker/lighter.
- I would like to have a perm (permanent wave).

Cars

As always, begin with key words. Clutch, brake, blinkers (*UK*, indicators), trunk (*UK*, boot), tank, gearbox, windshield (*UK*, windscreen) wipers, (steering) wheel, unleaded gas (*UK*, petrol), etc., must belong to your fund of knowledge of English, as well as several usual sentences such as:

- How far is the nearest gas (petrol) station? 20 miles from here.
- In what direction? Northeast/Los Angeles.

At the Gas/Petrol Station

- Fill it up, please.
- Unleaded, please.
- Could you jump-start my car battery, please?
- Could you check the oil, please?
- Could you check the tire pressure, please?
- Do you want me to check the spare tire too? Yes, please.
- Pump number 5, please.
- Can I have a receipt, please?

At the Garage

- My car has broken down.
- What do you think is wrong with it?
- Can you fix (*UK*, mend) a puncture?
- Can you take the car in tow to downtown Boston?
- I see …, kill the engine, please.
- Start the engine, please.
- The car goes to the right and overheats.
- Have you noticed if it loses water/gas/oil?
- Yes, it's losing oil.
- Does it lose speed?
- Yes, and it doesn't start properly.
- I can't get it into reverse.
- The engine makes funny noises.
- Please repair it as soon as possible.
- I wonder if you can fix it temporarily.
- How long will it take to repair?
- I am afraid we have to send for spare parts.
- The car is very heavy on petrol.
- I think the right front tire needs changing.
- I guess the valve is broken.
- Is my car ready?
- Have you finished fixing the car?
- Did you fix the car?
- Do you think you can fix it today?
- I think I've got a puncture rear offside.
- The spare's flat as well.
- I've run out of gas (*UK*, petrol).

At the Parking Lot (*UK*, Car *Park*)

- Do you know where the nearest car park is?
- Are there any free spaces?
- How much is it per hour?
- Is the car park supervised?
- How long can I leave the car here?

Renting a Car

- I want to rent a car. (*US*)
- I want to hire a car. (*UK*)
- For how many days?

- Unlimited mileage?
- What is the cost per mile?
- Is insurance included?
- You need to leave a deposit.

How Can I Get to ...?

- How far is Minneapolis?
- It is not far. About 12 miles from here.
- Is the road good?
- It is not bad, although a bit slow.
- Is there a toll road between here and Berlin?
- How long does it take to get to Key West?
- I am lost. Could you tell me how I can get back to the toll road.

Having a Drink (or Two)

Nothing is more desirable than a drink after a hard day of meetings. In such a relaxed situation embarrassing incidents can happen. Often, there is a difficult counter-question to a simple "Can I have a beer?" such as "Would you prefer lager?" or "small, medium, or large, sir?" From my own experience, when I was a beginner, I hated counter-questions and I remember my face flushing when, in a pub in London, instead of giving me the beer I asked for, the barman responded with the entire list of beers in the pub. "I have changed my mind, I'll have a Coke instead" was my response to both the "aggression" I suffered from the barman and the embarrassment resulting from my lack of fluency. "We don't serve Coke here, sir." These situations can spoil the most promising evening so ... let's review a bunch of usual sentences:

- Two beers please, my friend will pay.
- Two pints of bitter and half a lager, please.
- Where can I find a good place to go for a drink?
- Where can we go for a drink at this time of the evening?
- Do you know any pubs with live music?
- What can I get you?
- I'm driving. Just an orange juice, please.
- A glass of wine and two beers, please.
- A gin and tonic.
- A glass of brandy. Would you please warm the glass?
- Scotch, please.
- Do you want it neat, with water, or on the rocks?
- Make it a double.
- I'll have the same again, please.

- Two cubes of ice and a teaspoon, please.
- This is on me.
- What those ladies are having is on me.

On the Phone

Many problems start when you lift the receiver. You hear a continuous purring, different from the one you are used to in your country, or a strange sequence of rapid pips. Immediately, "what the hell am I supposed to do now" comes to your mind, and we face one of the most embarrassing situations for non-fluent speakers. The phone has two added difficulties: firstly, its immediacy and, secondly, the absence of images ("if I could see this guy I would understand what he was saying"). Do not worry; the preliminary exchanges in this conversational scenario are few. Answering machines are another, and tougher, problem and are out of the scope of this survival guide. Just a tip: do not hang up. Try to catch what the machine is saying and give it another try in case you are not able to follow its instructions. Many doctors, as soon as they hear the unmistakable sound of these devices, terrified, hang up thinking they are too much for them. Most messages are much easier to understand and less mechanical than those given by "human" (and usually bored) operators.

- Where are the public phones, please?
- Where is the nearest call-box?
- This telephone is out of order.
- Operator, what do I dial for the USA?
- Hold on a moment … number one.
- Would you get me this number please?
- Dial straight through.
- What time does the cheap rate begin?
- Have you got any phone cards, please?
- Can I use your cellular/mobile phone, please?
- Do you have a phone book (directory)?
- I'd like to make a reverse charge call to Korea.
- I am trying to use my phone card, but I am not getting through.
- Hello, this is Dr. Vida speaking.
- The line is busy (*UK*, engaged).
- There's noa nswer.
- It's a bad line.
- I've been cut off.
- I would like the number for Dr. Vida on Green Street.
- What is the area code for Los Angeles?
- I can't get through to this number. Would you dial it for me?
- Can you put me through to Spain?

Emergency Situations

- I want to report a fire/a robbery/an accident.
- This is an emergency. We need an ambulance/the police.
- Get me the police and hurry.

In the Bank

Nowadays, the spread of credit cards makes this section virtually unnecessary but, in my experience, when things go really wrong you may need to go to a bank. Fluency disappears in stressful situations so, in case you have to solve a bank problem, review not only this bunch of sentences but the entire section in your guide.

- Where can I change money?
- I'd like to change 200 Euros.
- I want to change 1000 Euros into Dollars/Pounds.
- Could I have it in tens, please?
- What's the exchange rate?
- What's the rate of exchange from Euros to Dollars?
- What are the banking hours?
- I want to change this travelers' check.
- Have you received a transfer from Rosario Nadal addressed to Fiona Shaw?
- Can I cash this bearer check?
- I want to cash this check.
- Do I need my ID to cash this bearer check?
- Go to the cash desk.
- Go to counter number 5.
- May I open a current account?
- Where is the nearest cash machine?
- I am afraid you don't seem to be able to solve my problem. Can I see the manager?
- Who is in charge?
- Could you call my bank in France? There must have been a problem with a transfer addressed to myself.

At the Police Station

- Where is the nearest police station?
- I have come to report a ...
- My wallet has been stolen.
- Can I call my lawyer (*UK*, solicitor)?

- I have been assaulted.
- My laptop has disappeared from my room.
- I have lost my passport.
- I will not say anything until I have spoken to my lawyer/solicitor.
- I have had a car accident.
- Why have you arrested me? I've done nothing.
- Am I under caution?
- I would like to call my embassy/consulate.

Printed in the United States
By Bookmasters